The American Board of Thoracic Surgery

A FIFTY YEAR PERSPECTIVE

Herbert Sloan, M.D.
Professor Emeritus of Surgery
University of Michigan Medical School
Ann Arbor, Michigan

Secretary-Treasurer
American Board of Thoracic Surgery
1973–1986

Printed in the United States of America.

ISBN 0-9626174-3-1

The American Board of Thoracic Surgery
One Rotary Center
Suite 803
Evanston, Illinois 60201

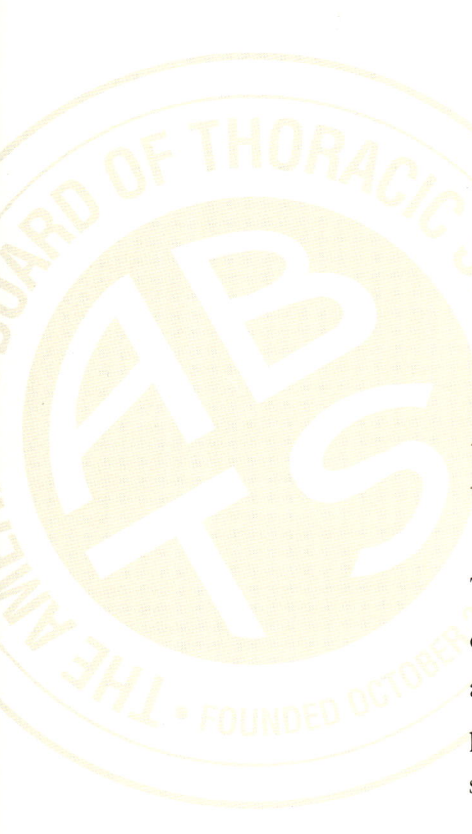

Dedication

This book is dedicated to Louise Sper who gave so much of herself to the Board and to all the Board members, past and present, who have worked to assure that the highest professional standards are maintained by cardiothoracic surgeons in the United States.

Foreword

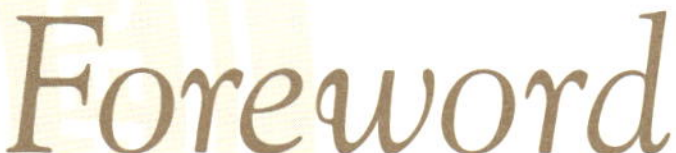

The second fifty years of the American Board of Thoracic Surgery are about to begin. Its history and solid foundation have been detailed by Herbert Sloan in a fashion that is both scholarly and readable. James Maloney has discussed the turbulent years when the Board relocated and went through many other changes in **Chapter 7**, and Richard Cleveland has outlined the Board's restructuring during the fifth decade, in **Chapter 8**.

The main function of the Board will always remain the certification examinations. The electronic age in which we function may, however, change the way the exam is given in the future.

Extensive discussion will continue as to whether or not certification in general surgery will remain as a requisite to sit for the thoracic examinations. Although there is considerable sentiment to shorten the length of residencies, no precipitous change will occur until a shorter pre-thoracic training residency is created that will be as good as or better than the one we have now.

The union of general thoracic and cardiac surgery will most likely continue. Board certified thoracic surgeons are relatively few in number and any separation would be counterproductive.

As new advances in thoracic surgery occur, the Board will react with changes in the so-called index case requirements. This will have to be done in conjunction with the Residency Review Committee (RRC).

Recertification will remain an essential, though voluntary, feature for thoracic surgery. Continued pressure from the government, managed care organizations, other third party payers, hospitals, and the public will continue to encourage the diplomate to maintain a valid certificate.

The next 50 years of the practice of thoracic surgery may not have the innovative excitement of the first five decades, but change and progress will continue. During this time, the American Board of Thoracic Surgery will continue to serve and protect the public by assuring that only those who are competent receive certification by passing both the written and oral examinations in thoracic surgery.

Marvin Pomerantz, M.D.
Chairman
American Board of Thoracic Surgery
1997–1999

Preface

As the American Board of Thoracic Surgery approaches the next century, it seems appropriate to review its first 50 years and try to record the people and events that shaped it. The Board and its staff have been the most important and rewarding part of my professional life.

Consideration of a thoracic board first surfaced seriously in 1936, but it was concluded that the time was not right. World War II increased the pressure to recognize thoracic surgery as a separate specialty and to create a certifying board. The Board of Thoracic Surgery was established in October 1948 as an Affiliate of the American Board of Surgery.

World War II also changed the lives of most of the young physicians who were entering medicine during those years, including my own. After a war shortened residency in general surgery and three years in the Armed Services, mostly spent in the Pacific, I began to seek further training and was interested in thoracic surgery. Dr. Max Chamberlain, one of the most charismatic people I have ever known, was responsible for getting me a residency in thoracic surgery at the University of Michigan.

In 1949 I took the second certifying examination given by the Board. That meant driving to Detroit where my written examination was to be administered in the Board Office. I got lost on the way but did have the opportunity of meeting Louise Sper for the first time. One of my examiners in Denver at the later oral examination was "Black" Tom Burford who was a most formidable presence. Later meetings with Bill Tuttle, the first Board Secretary, clearly put him in that same category.

As time went on, I had more contact with the Board and, finally, was elected a member. There then began a long series of associations with Board members, which made this experience so important and rewarding.

Not only was there the association with Board members, but there was the opportunity to work with Louise. This increased during my years as Secretary. She taught me a great deal, ran a very tight ship, and could solve any problem. She was meticulous and set high standards of performance that I was never able to meet. With the recognition and celebration of the Board's 50th anniversary, I regret so much that Louise Sper cannot be present to share it.

During these years it was my privilege to meet several of the original Board members who played such an important part in the creation and development of the Board. To a much younger person they were giants, but even as I age, they continue to be so. As time went on the Board faced increasing problems, which they met head on.

Examinations grew much more sophisticated, and the written examination changed to multiple choice questions with increasing emphasis on quality. The oral examination, originally highly individualistic, became more standardized. There was the mounting involvement in graduate medical education and its burgeoning bureaucracy. Finances were a serious problem that finally was solved with the establishment of an endowment supported by diplomates.

Although relations with the American Board of Surgery remained close, the thoracic board became a primary board and changed its name to the American Board of Thoracic Surgery. The Board dealt with the problem of cardiovascular surgery and supported it as a part of thoracic surgery. Finally, recertification was adopted, although not without considerable controversy. During all this time an extraordinary and ever-changing group of dedicated thoracic surgeons supported the Board's goals and worked hard to achieve them. The leadership of the chairmen was outstanding. Through it all, the Board reaffirmed repeatedly their purpose, to assure that thoracic surgeons certified by the Board were capable of providing safe care for their patients.

When Bob Shaw left the Board to work in Afghanistan, he was quoted and echoed by John Strieder as saying that the Board was the best "club" to which he had ever belonged. I can only support that statement.

Herbert Sloan, M.D.
Ann Arbor
August 1997

Acknowledgments

There are so many people who have contributed to the American Board of Thoracic Surgery and to this record that it is almost impossible to recognize them all. Nonetheless, some deserve special mention. First, of course, is Louise Sper who was the heart and soul of the Board almost from its beginning until her retirement in 1986. Her Recollections provided many of the personal notes recorded here. Louise died in Detroit on February 7, 1995. Louise's son, Leslie Sper, deserves our thanks for making available material and photographs Louise had collected and stored in her home.

Henry Bahnson, Rollin Daniel and Edward Beattie all contributed portions of Board history. George Humphreys added personal recollections of some of the first Board members.

An important contribution came from the personal correspondence of thoracic surgeons who had information about the Board and its beginnings. Among them were: Reeve Betts, Lewis Bosher, Lyman A. Brewer III, O. Theron Clagett, David Dugan, Julian Johnson, Hiram Langston, William Lees, Herbert Maier, Benson B. Roe, Paul Samson, and Robert Shaw.

Many individuals shared photographs from their personal collections, and we would like to thank and acknowledge them: David Dugan, Hans Ehrenhaft, Robert G. Ellison, Thomas B. Ferguson, George Humphreys, Frederick Kittle, George Magovern, James Malm, Donald Mulder, Hassan Najafi, W. Gerald Rainer, Benson B. Roe, Robert Shaw, Leslie Sper, and Myron Wheat.

James Maloney and Richard Cleveland provided enormous support by reviewing the first draft of the book and by contributing to bringing the Board history up-to-date. The manuscript was also reviewed by Edward Beattie, Robert Ellison, Thomas B. Ferguson, Glennis Lundberg, Hassan Najafi, and W. Gerald Rainer.

Finally, this history would never have been completed without the help and direction of Jeanne Fitzgerald who also helped me for so many years with the *Annals of Thoracic Surgery*. Working with her was Eloise Anagnost of ANAGraphics, who provided the attractive book design and graphic arts component of this history.

Table of Contents

Officers: Past & Present

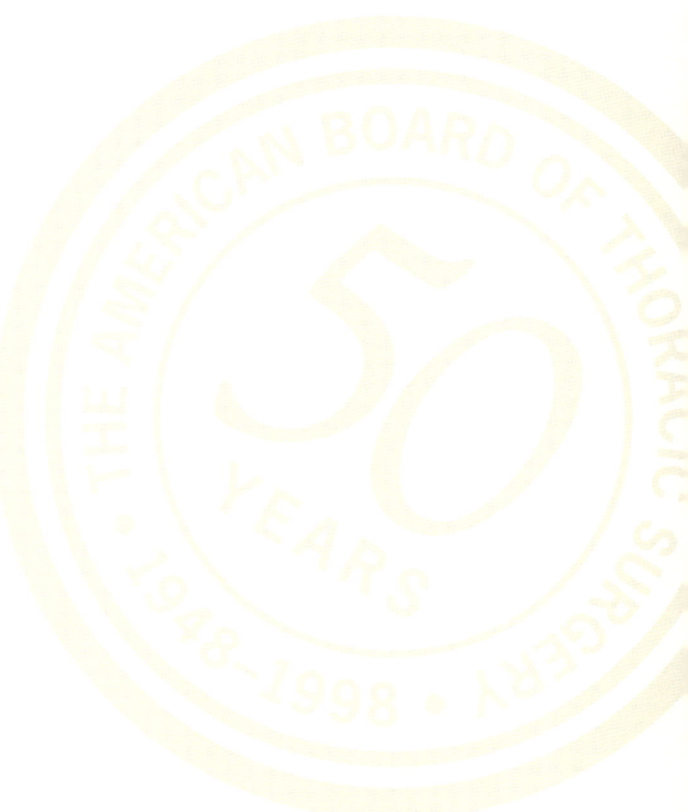

MEMBERS OF THE AMERICAN BOARD OF THORACIC SURGERY, 1948–1998

Current Officers

Marvin Pomerantz, M.D., *Chairman*
Fred A. Crawford, Jr., M.D., *Vice-Chairman*
Richard J. Cleveland, M.D., *Secretary-Treasurer*
Gordon F. Murray, M.D., *Examination Chairman*
Glennis Lundberg, *Administrative Director*

Current Directors

Richard P. Anderson, M.D.
William A. Baumgartner, M.D.
David P. Campbell, M.D.
James L. Cox, M.D.
Timothy J. Gardner, M.D.
Floyd D. Loop, M.D.
Douglas J. Mathisen, M.D.
Joseph I. Miller, Jr., M.D.
Gordon N. Olinger, M.D.
Peter C. Pairolero, M.D.
Carolyn E. Reed, M.D.
J. Kent Trinkle, M.D.

CURRENT OFFICERS OF THE BOARD

Chairman

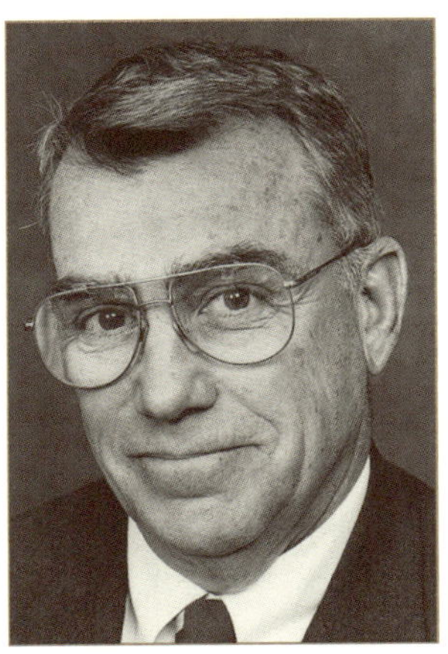

Marvin Pomerantz, M.D.
1997–1999

Vice-President

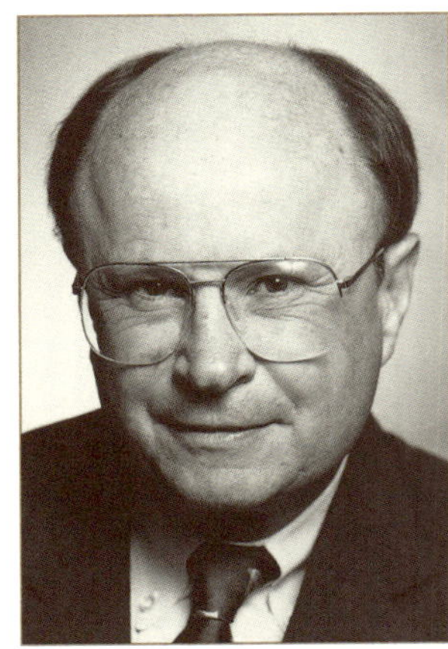

Fred A. Crawford, Jr., M.D.
1998–2000

Secretary-Treasurer

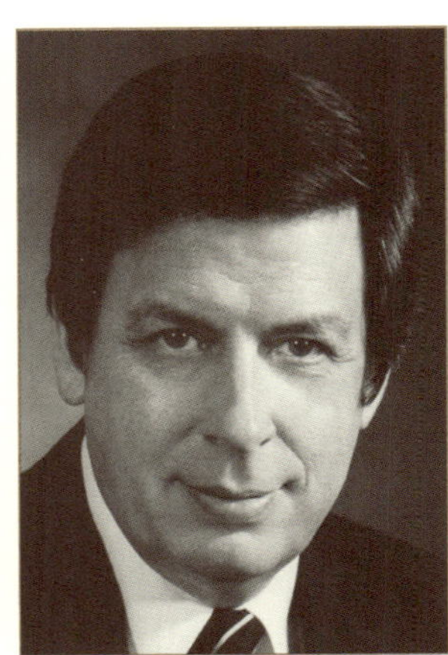

Richard J. Cleveland, M.D.
1991–1998

Examination Chairman

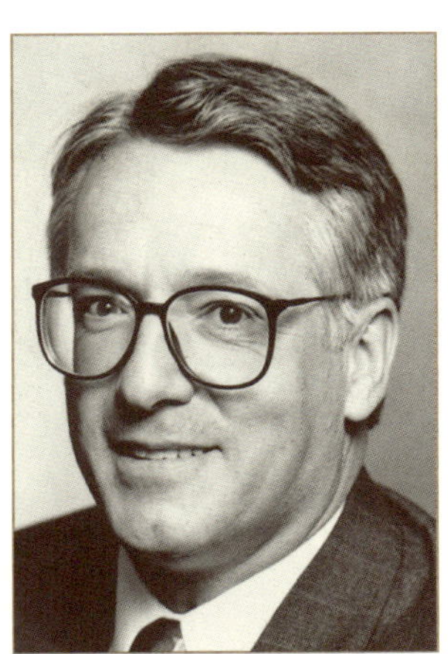

Gordon F. Murray, M.D.
1995–1998

Administrative Director

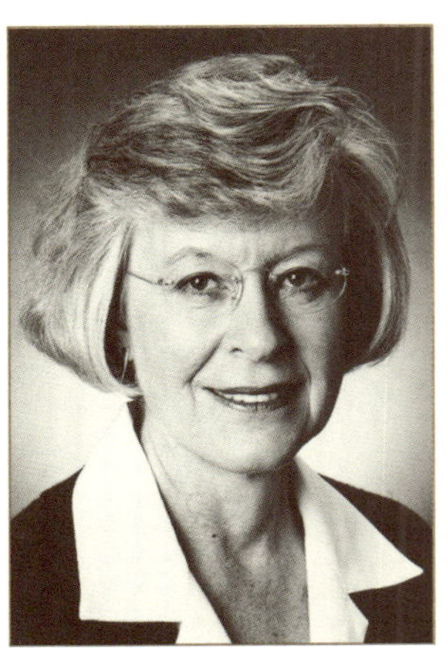

Glennis Lundberg
1986–1998

FORMER OFFICERS OF THE BOARD

Chairmen

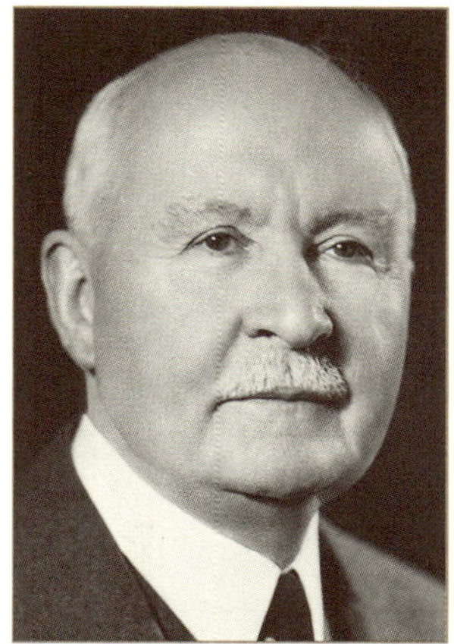
Carl Eggers, M.D.*
1948–1952

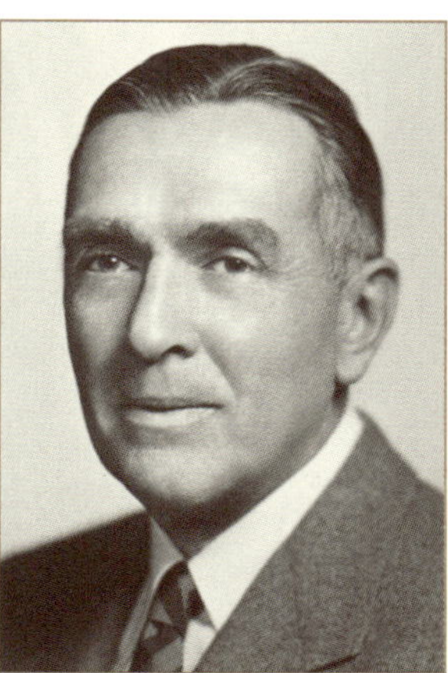
Cameron Haight, M.D.*
1952–1954

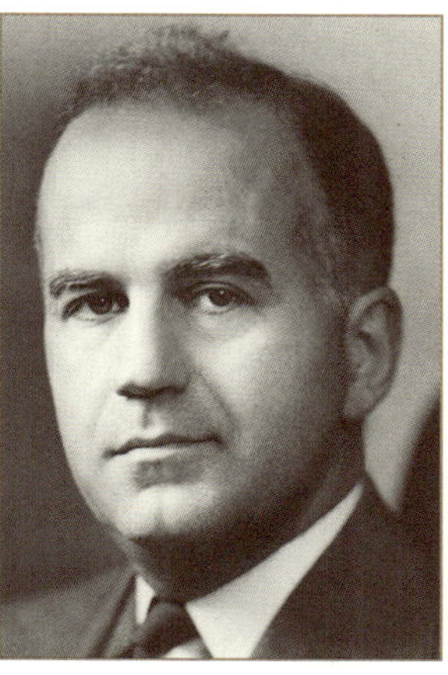
Richard H. Sweet, M.D.*
1954–1955

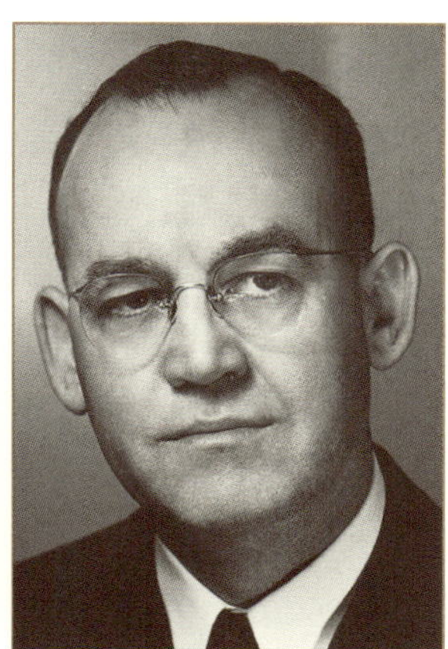
William E. Adams, M.D.*
1955–1957

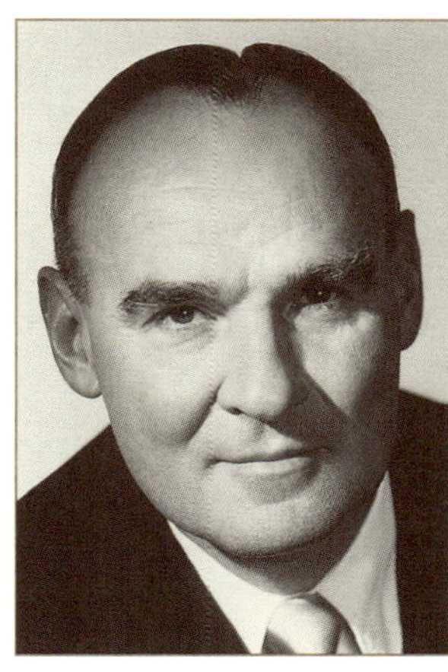
John C. Jones, M.D.*
1957–1959

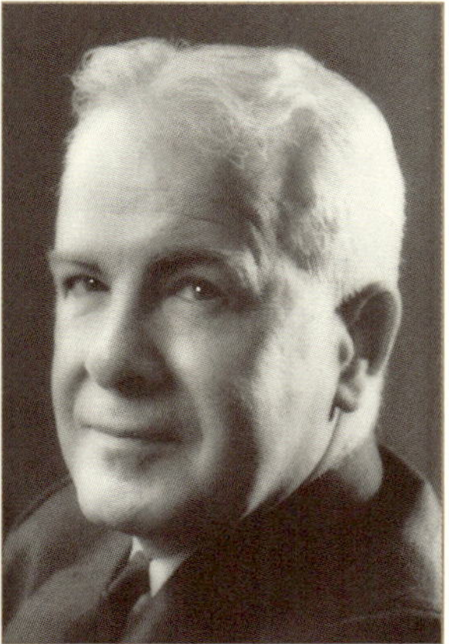
O. Theron Clagett, M.D.*
1959–1961

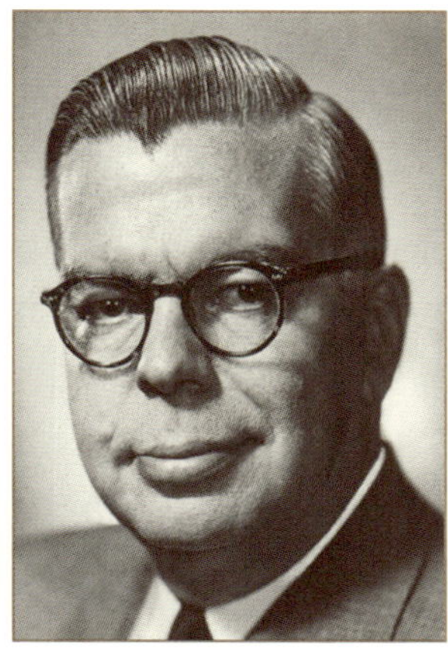
Herbert C. Maier, M.D.*
1961–1963

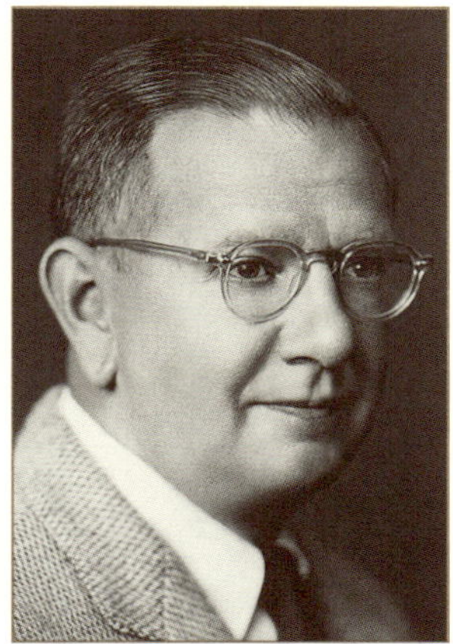
John W. Strieder, M.D.*
1963–1965

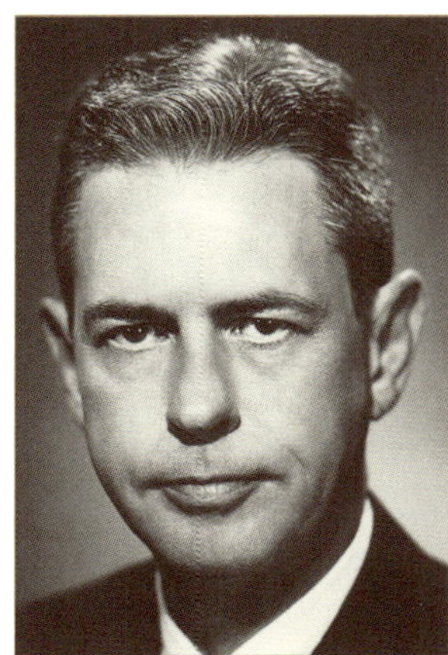
Rollin A. Daniel, Jr., M.D.*
1965–1967

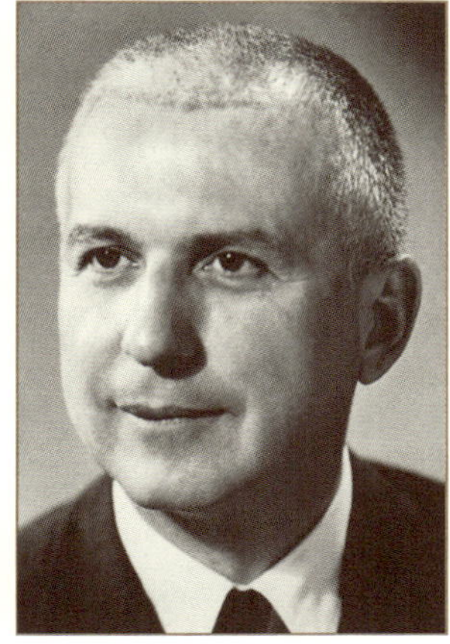
Edward J. Beattie, Jr., M.D.
1967–1969

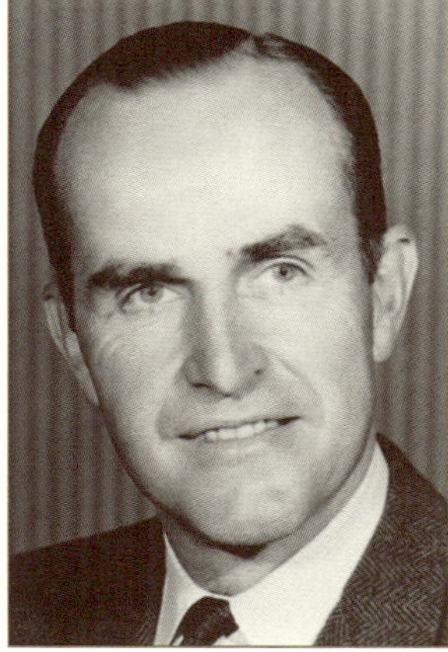
David J. Dugan, M.D.
1969–1971

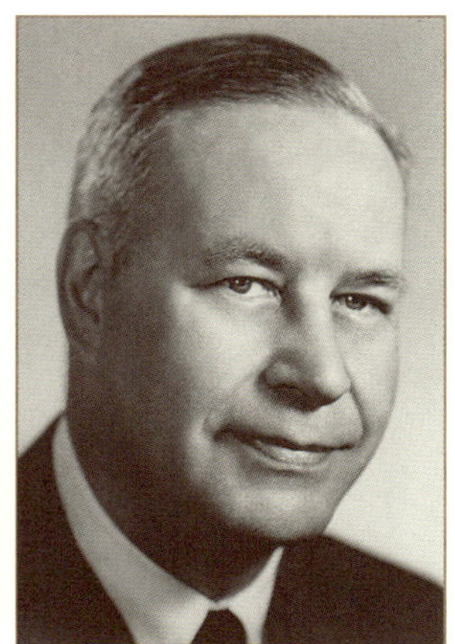
Donald L. Paulson, M.D.
1971–1973

FORMER OFFICERS OF THE BOARD

Chairmen *(continued)*

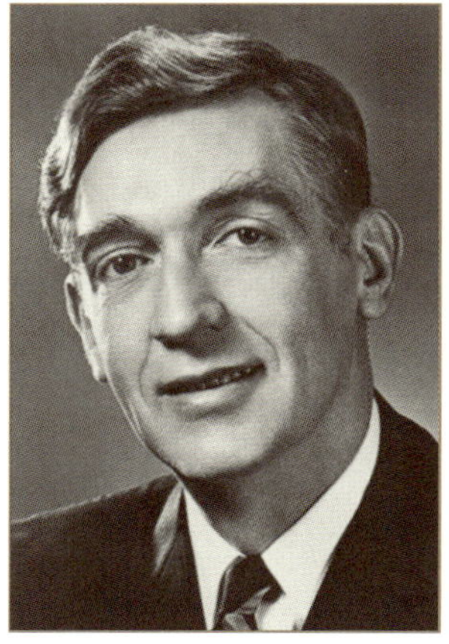
C. Frederick Kittle, M.D.
1973–1975

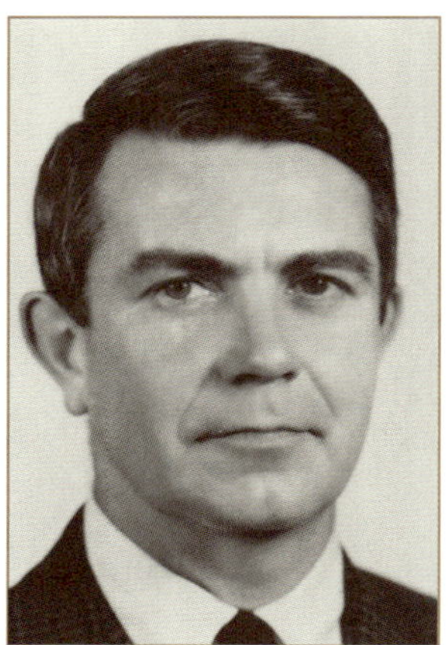
Paul C. Adkins, M.D.*
1975–1977

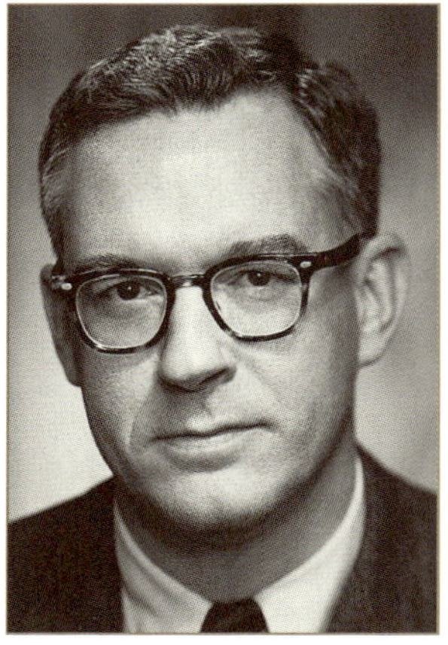
Thomas B. Ferguson, M.D.
1977–1979

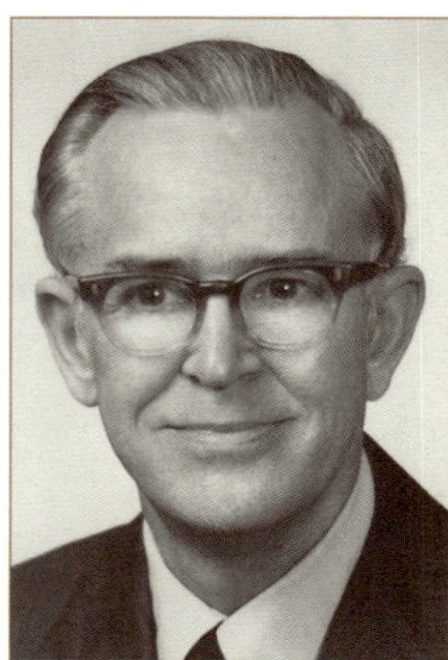
Robert G. Ellison, M.D.
1979–1981

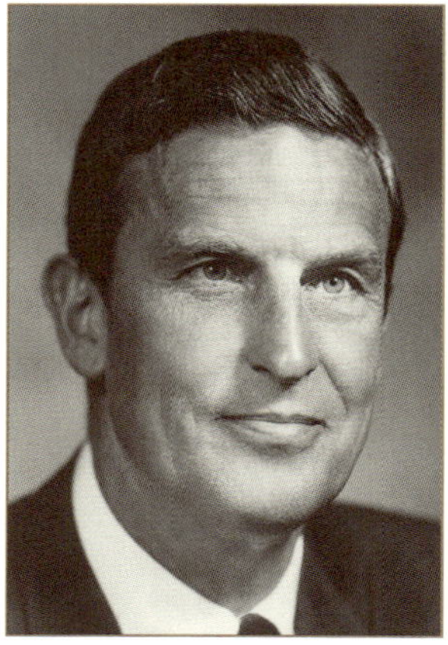
Benson B. Roe, M.D.
1981–1983

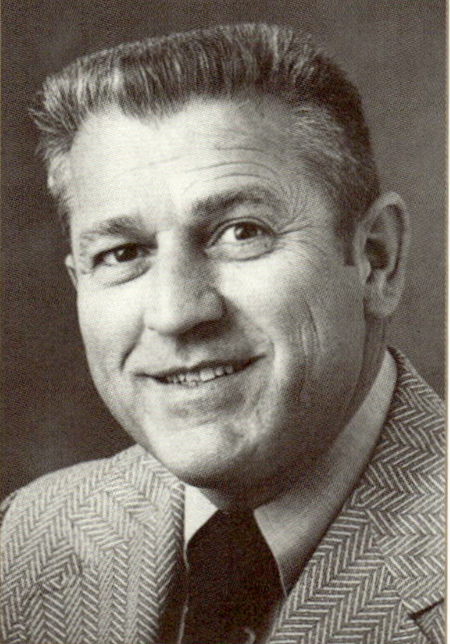
Donald G. Mulder, M.D.
1983–1985

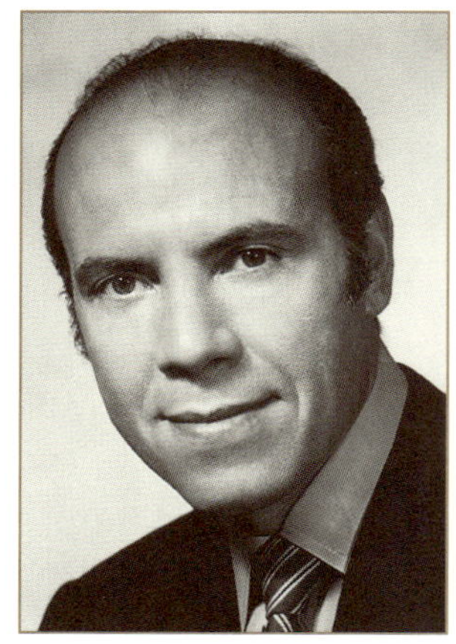
Hassan Najafi, M.D.
1985–1987

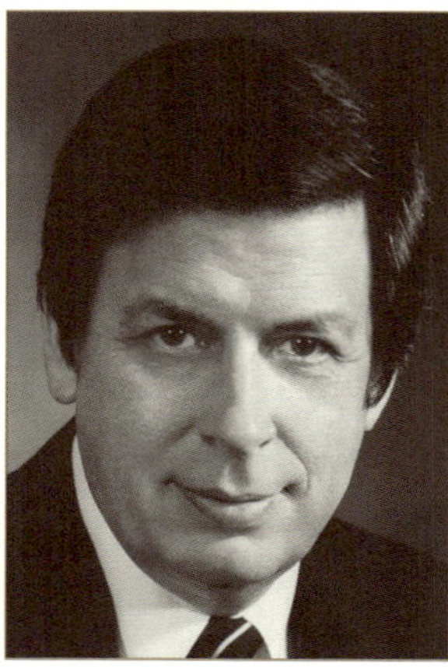
Richard J. Cleveland, M.D.
1987–1989

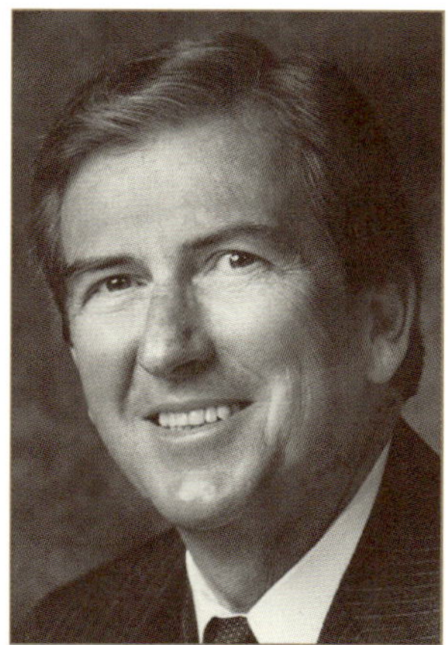
Harvey W. Bender, Jr., M.D.
1989–1991

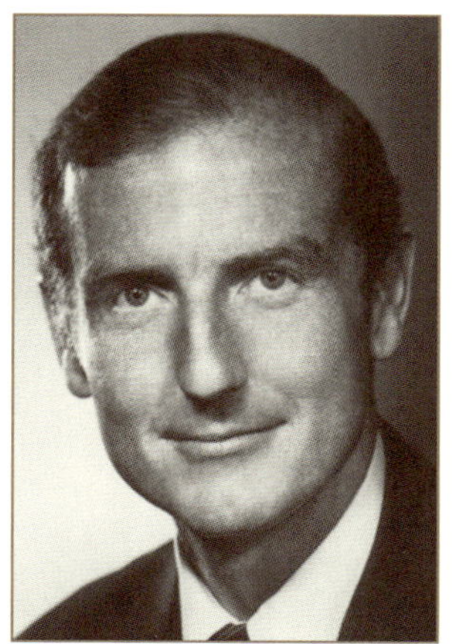
Benson R. Wilcox, M.D.
1991–1993

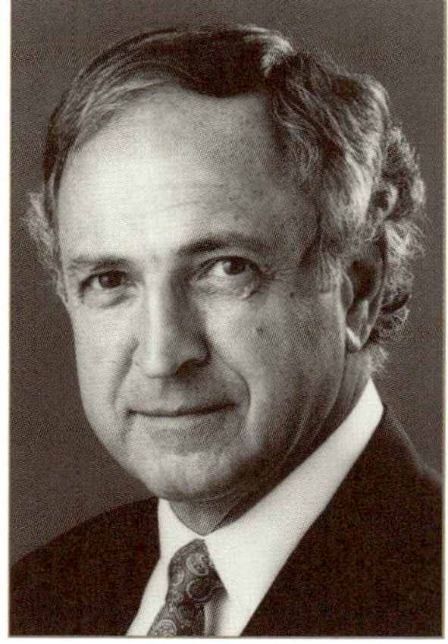
John Ochsner, M.D.
1993–1995

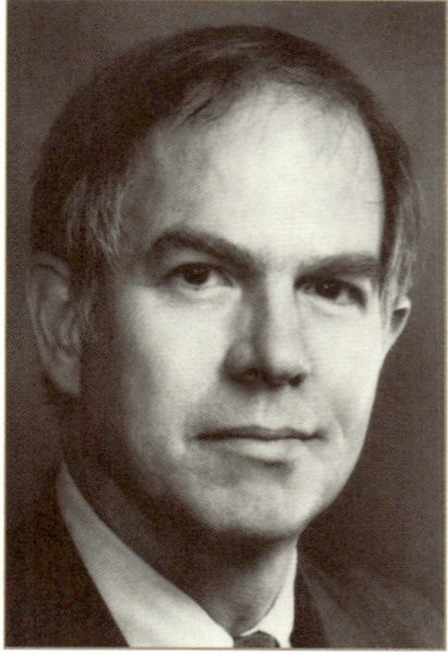
William A. Gay, Jr., M.D.
1995–1997

FORMER OFFICERS OF THE BOARD

Secretary-Treasurers

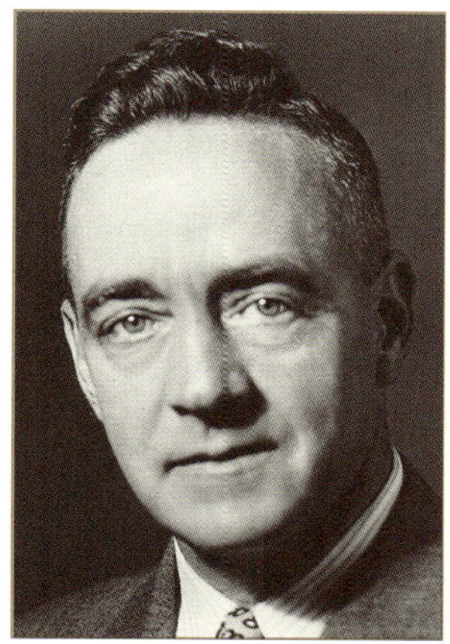

William M. Tuttle, M.D.*
1948–1962

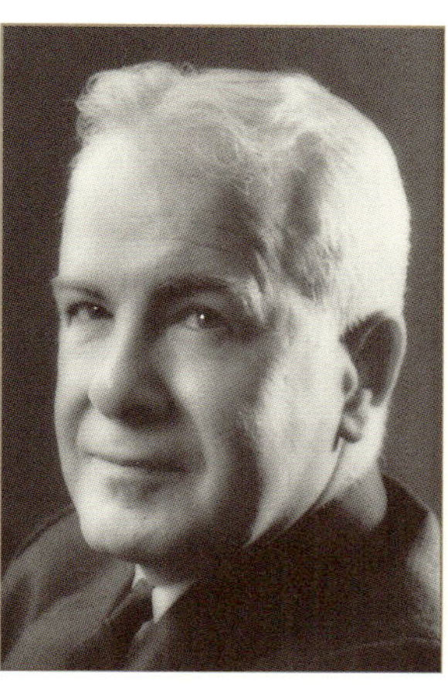

O. Theron Clagett, M.D.*
1963–1968

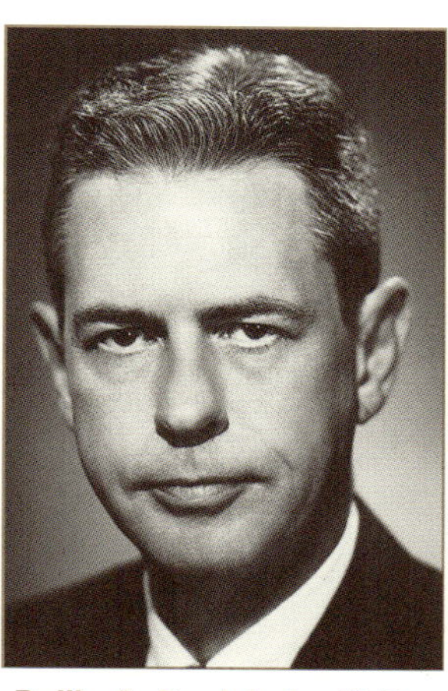

Rollin A. Daniel, Jr., M.D.*
1968–1973

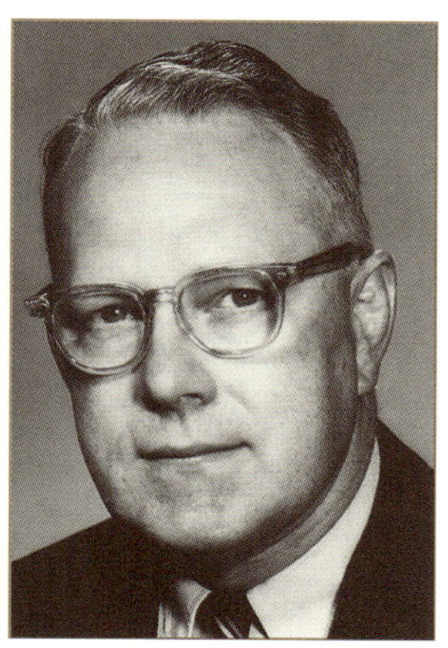

Herbert Sloan, M.D.
1973–1986

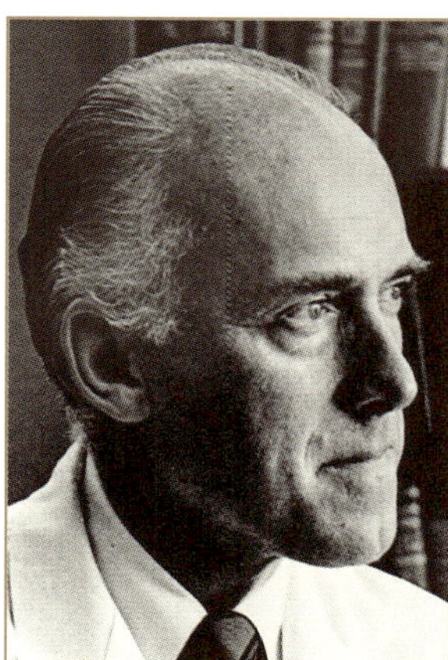

James V. Maloney, Jr., M.D.
1986–1991

FORMER OFFICERS OF THE BOARD

Vice-Chairmen

1948–1952	Cameron Haight, M.D.*
1952–1954	Richard H. Sweet, M.D.*
1954–1955	William E. Adams, M.D.*
1955–1957	John C. Jones, M.D.*
1957–1959	O. Theron Clagett, M.D.*
1959–1961	Herbert C. Maier, M.D.*
1961–1963	John W. Strieder, M.D.*
1963–1965	Rollin A. Daniel, Jr., M.D.*
1965–1967	Edward J. Beattie, Jr., M.D.
1967–1969	David J. Dugan, M.D.
1969–1971	Donald L. Paulson, M.D.
1971–1973	Herbert Sloan, M.D.
1973	C. Frederick Kittle, M.D.
1973–1975	Paul C. Adkins, M.D.*
1975–1977	Thomas B. Ferguson, M.D.
1977–1979	Robert G. Ellison, M.D.
1979–1981	Benson B. Roe, M.D.
1981–1983	Donald G. Mulder, M.D.
1983–1985	Hassan Najafi, M.D.
1985–1987	Richard J. Cleveland, M.D.
1987–1989	Paul A. Ebert, M.D.
1989–1991	Benson R. Wilcox, M.D.
1991–1993	John Ochsner, M.D.
1993–1995	William A. Gay, Jr., M.D.
1995–1997	Marvin Pomerantz, M.D.

Examination Chairman

1991–1994	L. Penfield Faber, M.D.

*Deceased

FORMER OFFICERS OF THE BOARD

Emeritus Directors of the Board

1948–1952	Carl Eggers, M.D.*
1948–1954	Cameron Haight, M.D.*
1948–1957	William E. Adams, M.D.*
1948–1953	Frank B. Berry, M.D.*
1948–1953	Brian B. Blades, M.D.*
1948–1955	Thomas H. Burford, M.D.*
1948–1955	Michael E. DeBakey, M.D.
1948–1952	Emile Holman, M.D.*
1948–1954	George H. Humphreys, M.D.
1948–1955	Richard H. Sweet, M.D.*
1952–1957	Julian Johnson, M.D.*
1953–1958	Joseph W. Gale, M.D.*
1953–1958	Paul C. Samson, M.D.*
1952–1959	John C. Jones, M.D.*
1954–1959	Robert H. Wylie, M.D.*
1955–1960	Edward M. Kent, M.D.*
1955–1960	Hiram T. Langston, M.D.*
1954–1961	O. Theron Clagett, M.D.*
1948–1962	William M. Tuttle, M.D.*
1955–1963	Herbert C. Maier, M.D.*
1957–1963	Robert R. Shaw, M.D.*
1958–1964	Anthony R. Curreri, M.D.*
1959–1965	Henry T. Bahnson, M.D.
1959–1965	Lyman A. Brewer, III, M.D.*
1957–1965	John W. Strieder, M.D.*
1960–1966	Paul W. Sanger, M.D.*
1958–1967	Rollin A. Daniel, Jr., M.D.*
1966–1968	Francis X. Byron, M.D.*
1960–1969	Edward J. Beattie, Jr., M.D.
1963–1969	Duane Carr, M.D.*
1963–1969	Donald B. Effler, M.D.
1965–1971	Denton A. Cooley, M.D.
1961–1971	David J. Dugan, M.D.
1965–1971	James V. Maloney, Jr., M.D.
1965–1971	J. Gordon Scannell, M.D.
1966–1972	Johann L. Ehrenhaft, M.D.
1964–1973	Donald L. Paulson, M.D.
1969–1975	Ralph D. Alley, M.D.*
1967–1975	C. Frederick Kittle, M.D.
1969–1975	Myron W. Wheat, Jr., M.D.
1969–1976	F. Henry Ellis, Jr., M.D.
1969–1976	James R. Malm, M.D.
1968–1977	Paul C. Adkins, M.D.*
1961–1977	Will C. Sealy, M.D.
1971–1978	Jay L. Ankeney, M.D.
1972–1978	Russell M. Nelson, M.D.
1973–1979	W. Sterling Edwards, M.D.
1969–1979	Thomas B. Ferguson, M.D.
1973–1979	Albert Starr, M.D.
1971–1981	Robert G. Ellison, M.D.
1975–1982	Harold C. Urschel, Jr., M.D.
1975–1982	Watts R. Webb, M.D.
1976–1982	John W. Kirklin, M.D.
1977–1983	Philip E. Bernatz, M.D.
1971–1983	Benson B. Roe, M.D.
1976–1983	Frank C. Spencer, M.D.
1978–1984	Hermes C. Grillo, M.D.
1978–1984	Quentin R. Stiles, M.D.
1979–1985	Harold V. Liddle, M.D.
1975–1985	Donald G. Mulder, M.D.
1979–1986	Charles R. Hatcher, Jr., M.D.
1966–1986	Herbert Sloan, M.D.

FORMER OFFICERS OF THE BOARD

Emeritus Directors of the Board *(continued)*

1977–1987	Hassan Najafi, M.D.
1986–1987	H. Edward Garrett, M.D.*
1982–1988	John R. Benfield, M.D.
1981–1988	Richard M. Peters, M.D.
1982–1988	W. Gerald Rainer, M.D.
1984–1988	W. Spencer Payne, M.D.
1982–1989	Paul A. Ebert, M.D.
1979–1989	Richard J. Cleveland, M.D.
1984–1990	W. Gerald Austen, M.D.
1983–1991	Harvey W. Bender, Jr., M.D.
1987–1991	James A. DeWeese, M.D.
1984–1991	George J. Magovern, M.D.
1985–1991	Martin F. McKneally, M.D.
1983–1993	Benson R. Wilcox, M.D.
1986–1994	L. Penfield Faber, M.D.
1986–1995	John Ochsner, M.D.
1988–1995	Mark B. Orringer, M.D.
1989–1995	John A. Waldhausen, M.D.
1989–1996	Nicholas J. Kouchoukos, M.D.
1990–1996	Mortimer J. Buckley, M.D.
1991–1996	Alden J. Harken, M.D.
1988–1997	William A. Gay, Jr., M.D.
1987-1993	Andrew S. Wechsler, M.D.

*Deceased

CHAPTER 1

The Beginnings

1925 National Board of Medical Examiners considers establishing a method of certifying individuals in the various specialties of medicine.

1936 Committee studies the problem of training thoracic surgeons with reference to certification by a national Board.

1937 Committee presents recommendations to AATS and newly formed American Board of Surgery.

A NEW IDEA GERMINATES

Early Discussions

The American Association for Thoracic Surgery (AATS) first discussed the certification of thoracic surgeons in 1925 when a letter was received from J. Stewart Rodman, then Secretary of the National Board of Medical Examiners. Two members of the Association were invited to meet with the National Board on May 6, 1925, to consider the value of establishing a method of certifying individuals in the various specialties of medicine. Dr. Rodman pointed out that no satisfactory method existed at that time to determine an individual's qualifications in many of the various specialty areas.

The invitation was read at the annual meeting of the Council of the American Association for Thoracic Surgery on May 3, 1925. It was accepted and Dr. Ethan Flagg Butler, long-time Secretary of the Association, and Dr. Robert T. Miller, Jr. were elected to represent the Association. Only Dr. Butler was able to attend the meeting; Dr. Miller was prevented from attending by an illness in his family.

AT THE PRESENT TIME (**1925**)...THERE IS NO UNIFORM METHOD OF DETERMINING THE QUALIFICATIONS OF GRADUATES IN MEDICINE TO ENGAGE IN THE PRACTICE OF THE SEVERAL SPECIALTIES IN MEDICINE AND SURGERY.

Dr. Butler reported back on the meeting to the Association. The Secretary of the National Board set forth the problem in this manner:

"At the present time (1925) there is ample provision, through the medical examiners of the several states and the National Board of Medical Examiners, for determining the primary qualifications of any graduate in medicine to engage in general practice. There is no uniform method of determining the qualifications of graduates in medicine to engage in the practice of the several specialties in medicine and surgery. The need for such certification is not clearly demonstrated as yet. Also, the practicality of such certification has not been clearly demonstrated."

Not surprisingly, considerable difference of opinion was expressed on the subject. The American Ophthalmological Association and the American Otolaryngological Association were already prepared to determine by examination whether or not individuals were qualified to practice these specialties, and they were prepared to issue certification of these qualifications. Other specialties were dubious about certification or felt it was desirable but questioned its practicality.

Dr. Butler expressed the opinion that, while he was in no way authorized to speak for the Association, it was his sense that the American Association for Thoracic Surgery believed certification was desirable. He also expressed the opinion that the Association, through its Council or its open meeting, would be glad to consider the question

1928 The first thoracic surgical training program begins as a two-year program.

1936 A questionnaire is sent to all AATS members prior to the annual meeting.

and candidly give its opinion to the National Board of Medical Examiners, provided this Board would place in the hands of the Association a questionnaire setting forth the points on which they desired information and discussion. In spite of this, the record indicates that no action was taken by the Association on this matter at that time, perhaps because there were too few thoracic surgeons and a prevailing belief that thoracic surgery was not yet a real specialty.

One of the first thoracic surgical training programs was established shortly after that in 1928 by Dr. John Alexander at the University of Michigan in Ann Arbor. In 1932 Dr. Alexander outlined his two year program of accepting students after the internship and two years of general surgical training.

THE SECOND WAVE

Questionnaire on Certification Sent

Prior to the Association's Annual Meeting in 1936, a questionnaire was sent to all AATS members, asking about thoracic surgery as a specialty (*see page 14*). The results of this questionnaire were included in the Presidential Address given by Dr. Eggers at the 1936 meeting of the Association. At this same meeting, Dr. Evarts Graham and Dr. John Alexander presented papers on the training of thoracic surgeons.[1,2,3]

---

1 Alexander, J., *Journal of Thoracic Surgery*, 1936; 5:579–582.
2 Eggers, C., *Journal of Thoracic Surgery*, 1936; 5:567–574.
3 Graham, E., *Journal of Thoracic Surgery*, 1936; 5:575–578.

169 questionnaires were sent out and 159 (94%) were returned. The breakdown of specialties was as follows:

1. General surgeons	97	61%
2. Thoracic surgeons	18	11%
3. Non-surgeons	44	27%

The responses were as follows:

1. Had special training in thoracic surgery:

a. General surgeons	34	35%
b. Thoracic surgeons	15	83%

2. Believed special training necessary or advantageous to practice thoracic surgery:

a. General surgery	91	94%
b. Thoracic surgeons	18	100%
c. Non-surgeons	39	89%

3. Believed it was preferable or sufficient to receive training during general surgery training:

a. General surgeons	59	61%
b. Thoracic surgeons	3	17%
c. Non-surgeons	13	30%

4. Believed thoracic surgery should be a defined specialty:

a. General surgeons	70	31%
b. Thoracic surgeons	17	95%
c. Non-surgeons	28	64%

5. Believed thoracic surgery should be practiced as a part of general surgery:

a. General surgeons	84	87%
b. Thoracic surgeons	3	17%
c. Non-surgeons	23	52%

Data gathered from the 1936 Questionnaire on Certification of Thoracic Surgeons.

"SOME FEEL IT IS NOW TIME FOR A SEPARATE SPECIALTY," NOTED DR. EGGERS. "OTHERS FEEL THORACIC SURGERY IS SAFEST IN THE HANDS OF GENERAL SURGEONS WITH A SPECIAL INTEREST IN THORACIC SURGERY."

Carl Eggers' presidential address was entitled, *Special Training for Thoracic Surgery*.[2] In it, Dr. Eggers noted that the purpose of the American Association for Thoracic Surgery was to solve problems related to surgery of the chest. Members included surgeons, internists, radiologists, endoscopists, and others interested in chest disease.

He also noted that thoracic surgery was the newest surgical specialty and that it was making rapid and spectacular progress. The question he posed was, "Where are we going?"

"Some feel it is now time for a separate specialty," noted Dr. Eggers. "Others feel thoracic surgery is safest in the hands of general surgeons with a special interest in thoracic surgery."

Dr. Eggers noted the bad results, particularly in the surgical treatment of tuberculosis. He pointed out that the questionnaire, which had been sent to the entire membership, had been developed to answer controversial points about specialization in thoracic surgery. Questions on the survey included:

- What specialties were represented in the respondent's experience and training?
- What training had the member received?
- What were the respondent's views about training?
- What were the respondent's views about specialization in thoracic surgery?

[2] Eggers, C., *Journal of Thoracic Surgery*, 1936; 5:567–574.

THORACIC SURGERY HAD BECOME COMPLEX, AND CONSISTENTLY GOOD RESULTS COULD BE OBTAINED ONLY BY SURGEONS WITH SPECIAL KNOWLEDGE OF THORACIC DISEASE AND BROAD, PRACTICAL EXPERIENCE WITH SURGERY OF THE CHEST.

Dr. Eggers concluded by stating that there was overwhelming opinion that special training in thoracic surgery was necessary. All agreed that good training in general surgery was necessary as well. He believed the problem of a separate specialty for thoracic surgery would resolve itself as time went on. Dr. Eggers doubted that the members of the Association were ready to separate thoracic surgery from general surgery.

Alexander and Graham Voice Opinions

John Alexander's paper, entitled *The Training of a Surgeon Who Expects to Specialize in Thoracic Surgery*, made the following points:

1. Many thoracic operations were being performed by surgeons with little training.
2. Thoracic surgery had become complex, and consistently good results could be obtained only by surgeons with special knowledge of thoracic disease and broad, practical experience with surgery of the chest.
3. Fewer than two years of intensive training in a very active thoracic surgical clinic were insufficient.
4. A two year program of graduated responsibility had been established at the University of Michigan, Ann Arbor, in 1928, and he went on to describe it.

DR. GRAHAM POINTED OUT THAT, IN 1917 WHEN THE AMERICAN ASSOCIATION FOR THORACIC SURGERY WAS FORMED, NOT ONE MEMBER CONSIDERED HIMSELF A SPECIALIST IN THORACIC SURGERY.

5. Interestingly, he spoke about the need for residents to have good health and a suitable temperament and personality. (I wonder how he would have described those characteristics.) Dr. Alexander also suggested that the resident have a reading knowledge of German with an added benefit being the ability to read French, Italian, and Spanish.

Evarts Graham's paper was titled, *Training of the Thoracic Surgeon from the Standpoint of the General Surgeon.*[3] This paper questioned whether or not thoracic surgery is a separate branch of surgery that may require special qualifications but also emphasized that sound training in general surgery is necessary.

Dr. Graham pointed out that, in 1917 when the American Association for Thoracic Surgery was formed, not one member considered himself a specialist in thoracic surgery. In 1936 there were a few members who considered themselves specialists in thoracic surgery, and he predicted that later there would be many such individuals.

Noting that he was chairman of a committee to consider the formation of an American Board of Surgery, Dr. Graham described some of the ways in which the Board might function:

[3] Graham, E., *Journal of Thoracic Surgery*, 1936; 5:575–578.

1936 AATS President appoints certification committee to study the question of training for thoracic surgeons.

1937 Certification Study Committee presents report at the AATS annual meeting in Chicago, Illinois.

1. He suggested that it was probably not desirable for certification of thoracic surgeons to be entirely separate from general surgery.
2. He also suggested that certification in general surgery should precede certification in thoracic surgery.
3. Finally, Dr. Graham suggested that the American Association for Thoracic Surgery might establish a special committee to consider the problem of thoracic surgical certification.

CERTIFICATION STUDY COMMITTEE APPOINTED

When the subject of certification arose again in 1936, the President of the Association appointed a committee to study the problem of the training of thoracic surgeons, with particular reference to their certification by a national board. The members of the committee were:

John Alexander
Edward W. Archibald
Edward D. Churchill
Daniel C. Elkin
Leo Eloesser
Evarts A. Graham
Carl Eggers, *Chairman*

The report of that committee was given during the 1937 AATS meeting at the Palmer House in Chicago, and in that report were four resolutions which were adopted and later accepted by the Association.

1937 The AATS committee meets on May 30 in Saranac Lake, New York, and approves the report and resolutions.

These were:

1. Be it resolved that the American Association for Thoracic Surgery recognize the American Board of Surgery as the parent organization which should properly be in control of all matters pertaining to the training and certification of surgeons and surgical specialists.
2. Be it further resolved that the American Association for Thoracic Surgery signify to the American Board of Surgery its willingness to cooperate with it, if and when the special certification of thoracic surgeons seems desirable.
3. Be it further resolved that, in case a subcommittee be desired by the American Board of Surgery, it be appointed by the Council of the AATS and that it be composed of surgical members of the Association.
4. The function of the subcommittee should be determined by the American Board of Surgery.

The American Board of Surgery, which was then in the process of formation, met in Chicago at the same time and permitted a joint meeting of the two committees later in the day. After developing its report, the AATS committee joined members of the American Board of Surgery for the combined meeting and presented its resolutions. The AATS committee stated that the resolutions would first have to be passed by the Association at its meeting before becoming official. The AATS committee had a second meeting on Sunday, May 30, 1937, at the home of Dr. Edward S. Welles of Saranac Lake, New York, at

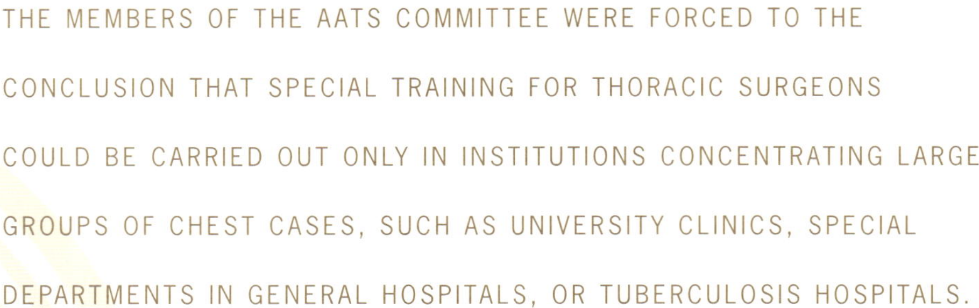
THE MEMBERS OF THE AATS COMMITTEE WERE FORCED TO THE CONCLUSION THAT SPECIAL TRAINING FOR THORACIC SURGEONS COULD BE CARRIED OUT ONLY IN INSTITUTIONS CONCENTRATING LARGE GROUPS OF CHEST CASES, SUCH AS UNIVERSITY CLINICS, SPECIAL DEPARTMENTS IN GENERAL HOSPITALS, OR TUBERCULOSIS HOSPITALS.

which time the report and resolutions were approved by the Council for adoption by the Association.

The report included data about numbers of thoracic surgeons and training programs. For example, in 1936, only 18 members of the Association had characterized themselves as specialists in thoracic surgery and had restricted their work to that specialty. In addition, there were only 24 thoracic surgical residencies in existence. This information was gathered through a questionnaire that had been sent to members of the Association earlier that same year (*see page 14*). Several additional findings had emerged:

1. Most importantly, the majority of the members of the Association, who were general surgeons with a special interest in thoracic surgery, were opposed to having a resident in thoracic surgery.
2. The average general hospital did not have a sufficient number of chest cases to warrant a resident in thoracic surgery.
3. Even if there was sufficient clinical material, it was deemed to be so scattered that it would not be available for teaching.

The members of the AATS committee were forced to the conclusion that special training for thoracic surgeons could be carried out only in institutions concentrating large groups of chest cases, such as university clinics, special departments in general hospitals, or tuberculosis hospitals.

THE COMMITTEE PUT ITSELF ON RECORD AS STANDING OPPOSED TO THE FURTHER SPLITTING UP OF GENERAL SURGERY INTO SUBDIVISIONS.

The committee then considered the question of establishing a special certifying board for thoracic surgery. They found that several surgical specialties had certifying boards. These included general surgery, gynecology, urology, otolaryngology, ophthalmology, and orthopedic surgery. In addition to these, a number of other surgical specialties might eventually claim recognition as independent specialties and desire their own certifying boards.

The committee put itself on record as standing opposed to the further splitting up of general surgery into subdivisions. They proposed that the American Association for Thoracic Surgery recognize the principle that all surgeons, whatever their interests, be trained as general surgeons. The key points were:

1. All future thoracic surgeons must be well trained general surgeons, as determined by the American Board of Surgery.
2. General surgeons will of necessity continue to perform thoracic operations as far as their ability and inclinations permit.
3. For those who desire to prepare themselves as thoracic surgeons, special opportunities for training must be provided.
4. Such training may be of a longer or shorter period. It was possible to visualize a short period of training to supplement the training of a young general surgeon. It was also possible to visualize a long period of training of two or more years to include all technical procedures used in the diagnosis and treatment of thoracic disease. Such residencies or fellowships would qualify the trainee to become a specialist.

THE **1937** REPORT OF THE AATS COMMITTEE, REPRESENTS THE STARTING POINT FOR THE ESTABLISHMENT OF A CERTIFYING BOARD FOR THORACIC SURGERY.

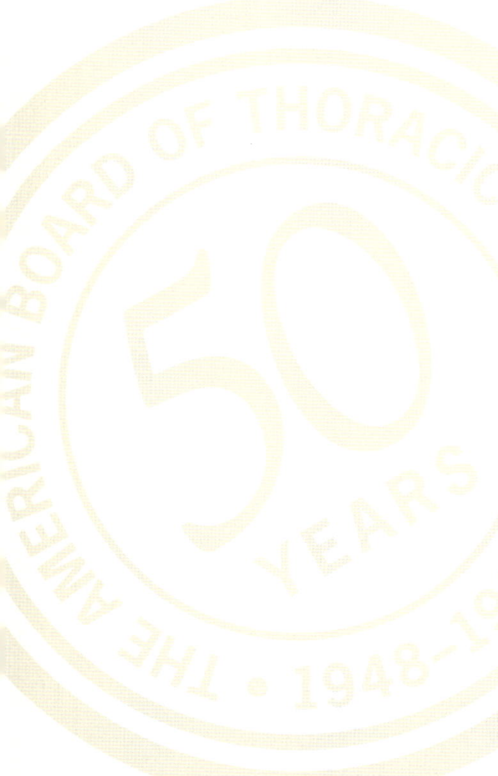

The committee felt it would not be wise for the Association to stray too far from the purposes for which it was founded. Thus, they did not recommend to the Association the establishment of its own certifying board, but rather, favored cooperation with the American Board of Surgery. Of the members of the committee, only John Alexander was in favor of establishing a thoracic board at that time.

The 1937 report of that AATS committee, represents the starting point for the establishment of a certifying board for thoracic surgery, even though they decided against doing it then. The members of the committee were among the most senior members of the Association and undoubtedly represented its most mature thinking.

A number of factors influenced the Association's decision: The American Board of Surgery was just being formed. Most surgical members of the Association were general surgeons with special interests in thoracic surgery, but relatively few limited their practice to thoracic surgery. Even after the formation of the Board of Thoracic Surgery, close ties with the American Board of Surgery remained. A fundamental principle of thoracic training has always been excellent training in general surgery before embarking on thoracic training.

THE IMPACT OF WORLD WAR II

World War II awakened interest in certification for thoracic surgeons again. In the military system certification meant higher rank and more pay. The Army, at least, did not recognize thoracic surgery as a specialty

1940–1945 During World War II, thoracic surgery matures. Surgeons in the field increase pressure to certify thoracic surgeons.

1943 The first Chest Surgery Center of the Armed Forces was established at Bizerte, Tunisia, during the North African campaign of World War II.

early in the war. One well trained thoracic surgeon was assigned to the septic ward at a general hospital in the United States because, "In World War I, empyema was the only thoracic condition treated."

Thoracic surgery matured during World War II. Perhaps this is best illustrated by the thoracic surgeons in the Second Auxiliary Surgical Group located first in the Mediterranean theater. These surgeons collected material on 2,267 thoracic casualties treated by thoracic surgical teams in the group. Their data demonstrated what careful and systematic planning could accomplish even under the stress of battle.

The first Chest Surgery Center of the Armed Forces was established at Bizerte, Tunisia, during the North African campaign in 1943. Among the men responsible for this were Drs. Thomas Burford, Lyman Brewer, and Paul Samson who, with others in the group, returned after the War to lead thoracic surgery in this country. The maturation of thoracic surgery in the Armed Forces is carefully recorded in two volumes published by the Medical Department of the United States Army. These volumes record the tremendous advances made in the treatment of thoracic injuries during the war.

The young thoracic surgeons in the North African theater of operations wrote frequent letters to their mentors in this country complaining about the lack of recognition of thoracic surgery, particularly when specialties such as orthopedics and neurosurgery were well established. These concerns, as well as medical problems, were

1946 Dr. Robert Shaw, who had been in the European theater, raises the question of recognition of thoracic surgery as a specialty in a letter to Dr. Alexander.

extensively discussed around the pot-bellied stoves needed to dispel the cold of the African nights. The intellectual climate was greatly improved, it is said, by the use of a mixture of hospital alcohol and grapefruit juice known as *yaki docky*.

At the close of World War II in 1945, Reeve Betts, a member of the Second Auxiliary, wrote J. Stewart Rodman, then Secretary of the American Board of Surgery, asking about the progress that had been made in recognizing thoracic surgery as a specialty. Dr. Rodman replied that it was his personal belief that the American Board of Surgery would be sympathetic to the idea.

In 1946 Dr. Robert Shaw, who had been in the European theater, wrote to Dr. Alexander, raising the question of recognition of thoracic surgery as a specialty. Dr. Shaw spoke bitterly about a consultant surgeon in the European Theater of Operations who said, "The only difference between a thoracic surgeon and a general surgeon was that the former drained through a stiff rubber tube and the latter through a soft tube." He also noted that, because of its lack of specialty recognition, thoracic surgery was a foster child under the consultant in plastic surgery in the European Theater.

CHAPTER 2

The Board Is Born

1946 Original certification study committee is reappointed; committee recommends formation of a Board.

1946 The Association adopts a formal resolution recommending the formation of a Board of Thoracic Surgery.

THE RESOLUTION

In 1945 and the early part of 1946 there was an interesting exchange of letters between Dr. Evarts Graham, Dr. John Alexander, and Dr. Carl Eggers. Having heard from the young thoracic surgeons who served in World War II about the need for recognition of thoracic surgery as a specialty, they decided that steps should be taken to organize an examining board for thoracic surgery.

In 1945 John Alexander stated to Evarts Graham, "I hope and believe that both the American Board of Surgery and the Advisory Board for Medical Specialties would, in equity, approve a Board for thoracic surgery, since it is perhaps the only specialty not represented by a Board."

Dr. Graham responded affirmatively, although he also stated that he saw some impediments to formation of a separate board, including the fact that many key figures such as Dr. Churchill, were still not discharged from the Army. He noted that the Advisory Board for Medical Specialties would first have to be approached on the idea of a separate thoracic board before any further action could be taken. Dr. Eggers also wrote to Dr. Alexander in 1946 about the desire of the

IN **1945** JOHN ALEXANDER STATED TO EVARTS GRAHAM, "I HOPE AND BELIEVE THAT BOTH THE AMERICAN BOARD OF SURGERY AND THE ADVISORY BOARD FOR MEDICAL SPECIALTIES WOULD...APPROVE A BOARD FOR THORACIC SURGERY..."

younger thoracic surgeons for a Board and the reactivation of the AATS committee formed in 1936 to consider the question of a Board once more.

In 1945 the President of the Association, Dr. Claude Beck, reappointed the original Committee to bring a report to the next meeting. At this 1946 meeting, the Committee made its report and the Association adopted a formal resolution recommending the formation of a Board of Thoracic Surgery.

The Vote

At the 1947 meeting of the Association, the members voted to accept the proposals of the American Board of Surgery for the establishment of a subsidiary Board of Thoracic Surgery. At the previous meeting, the Association had voted to enter into negotiations with the American Board of Surgery for the establishment of such a subsidiary Board. The Committee acting for the Association was composed of: Dr. Carl Eggers, Chairman, Dr. Jerome Head, and Dr. Alton Ochsner. The Association authorized the President, Dr. Alton Ochsner, and the Council to continue negotiations with the Committee of the American Board of Surgery for the purpose of:

1. Organizing the Board of Thoracic Surgery.
2. Establishing a founders group.
3. Appointing an examining committee.
4. Setting up requirements for training and certification of thoracic surgeons.

1947 AATS approves establishment of affiliate Board of Thoracic Surgery

Further Negotiations; Another Questionnaire

Following the 1947 meeting, the current AATS President, Dr. Edward Churchill, appointed the following committee to continue negotiations with the American Board of Surgery: Dr. Carl Eggers, Chairman, Dr. I. A. Bigger, Dr. Brian Blades, Dr. Cameron Haight and Dr. Richard H. Meade, Jr. Within the ensuing year, Dr. Bigger resigned from the Committee and was replaced by Dr. Dan Elkin. During that year Herbert Maier was also added to the Committee.

During this time period a second questionnaire, similar to the first one in 1936, was circulated among the 200 members of the Association. Of these, 150 (75%) returned the questionnaire: 87 general surgeons with a special interest in thoracic surgery and 45 individuals describing themselves as specialists in thoracic surgery:

The tally of responses revealed the following:

	Yes	No
Favor special training in thoracic surgery:	Yes (133)	No (2)
Thoracic surgery should be a specialty:	Yes (112)	No (17)
Thoracic surgeons should be certified:	Yes (114)	No (17)

The change in responses from the previous questionnaire in 1936 is striking. Greater numbers of surgeons were specializing in thoracic surgery, and there was much wider acceptance of thoracic surgery as a specialty, together with the desire for a certifying process. One handwritten note, probably from Dr. Herbert Maier, included a statement

GREATER NUMBERS OF SURGEONS WERE SPECIALIZING IN THORACIC SURGERY, AND THERE WAS MUCH WIDER ACCEPTANCE OF THORACIC SURGERY AS A SPECIALTY, TOGETHER WITH THE DESIRE FOR A CERTIFYING PROCESS.

that the candidate, "shall likewise have had a satisfactory period of training in bronchoscopy and esophagoscopy."

THE PROPOSAL

The report to the Association at their 1948 meeting discussed at length the proposed relationship with the American Board of Surgery and the meaning of thoracic surgery becoming a specialty. Additional discussion considered specialist training and the ways in which it might be achieved. Finally, a proposed plan of organization was presented. Key points included:

1. *Name*. This topic provoked debate as to whether to call the organization the Board of Thoracic Surgery or the American Board of Thoracic Surgery. For the time being, the name Board of Thoracic Surgery was chosen.
2. *Organization*. The cooperating national surgical societies elected jointly to form the Board with the following representation:
    - The American Association for Thoracic Surgery: 4 members
    - The American Surgical Association: 3 members
    - The American College of Surgeons: 2 members
    - The Surgical Section of the American Medical Association: 2 members

A rotating term of membership by the stagger system was established with each term lasting five years. The Secretary would serve for a longer, as yet indeterminate number of years.

1948 The formation of the Board progresses with an organizational meeting held in Detroit, Michigan on October 2.

1949 Training requirements are established. Examination to be written, oral, and practical. First written and oral examinations are administered.

3. *Constitution and Bylaws*. These articles were the same as for the American Board of Surgery.
4. *Qualification Requirements for Applicants*. These included:
   a. Certification by the American Board of Surgery.
   b. Two years training in thoracic surgery in institutions approved by the Board of Thoracic Surgery, or meritorious contributions to thoracic surgery.
   c. Successful completion of written, oral, and practical examinations. (In fact, the practical examination was never administered.)
5. *Definition of Acceptable Training in Thoracic Surgery*. To qualify for the examination in thoracic surgery, the candidate must have had two years of training in an active, well-integrated, thoracic surgical clinic or clinics, or the equivalent amount of thoracic surgical training on a mixed service consisting of thoracic and nonthoracic surgical cases. The training was to consist of adequate preparation in both the tuberculous and non-tuberculous aspects of thoracic surgery. Under exceptional circumstances certain surgeons could, by virtue of recognized proficiency in the surgical treatment of thoracic disease, qualify for the examination at the discretion of the Board.
6. *Founders Group*. This body was to be composed of surgeons who had made meritorious contributions to thoracic surgery, as follows:
   a. Active and senior members of the American Association for Thoracic Surgery, already certified by the American Board of Surgery, were to become founder members, automatically.

DIFFERENCES OF OPINION PERSISTED FOR MANY YEARS, PARTICULARLY IN THE AREA OF CARDIAC SURGERY WHERE THE TURF BATTLES WERE ESPECIALLY HARD FOUGHT.

b. Other surgical members of the American Association for Thoracic Surgery would have their records reviewed by the Board, and could be recommended for Founder Membership with or without application.
c. Other surgeons, certified by the American Board of Surgery who, upon application, and after review of their qualifications, could be found to meet the requirements of the Board. A number of names for the Founders Group were submitted at that time. The Founders Group would then be kept open for two years after organization of the Board.

7. *Group to be Certified by Examination.* Only candidates who had been certified by the American Board of Surgery would be eligible for examination.

The Board of Thoracic Surgery would review the candidate's training or accomplishments in thoracic surgery. If acceptable, he would be notified to appear for examination.

In the report there was discussion of opportunities for training in thoracic surgery, and it suggested that opportunities for training had increased significantly. It was also recommended that the examination process would be governed by the rules laid down by the American Board of Surgery, although the Board of Thoracic Surgery would retain the right to change the rules. For the Founders Group,

1949 The Board establishes its home at the Herman Kiefer Hospital in Detroit, Michigan.

1950 The State of Michigan grants corporate charter.

the fee would be $25.00. For candidates to be certified by examination the fee would be $50.00.

The proposal to create a Board of Thoracic Surgery was not greeted with uniform enthusiasm. Dr. Churchill himself wrote the following:

"Of course, I really wish the boys would give up the idea of having this special Board. Their chief idea seems to be to stop some sanatorium superintendents from doing thoracoplasties, but a Board is not going to accomplish this. There are not enough people to do the thoracoplasties anyway.

"I do not see how anyone has the temerity to call himself a thoracic surgeon in these days. The chest is a busy place, and the neurosurgeons are after the sympathetic trunk, the abdominal surgeons after the stomach and spleen, and fellows like Al Blalock and Bob Gross are playing with the heart.

"Just how any one fellow thinks he has the proficiency to do all these better than anyone else is more than I can see. A few years ago when we were concerned with collapse for tuberculosis and a few cases of cutting out of the lung, or part of the lung, it was a different matter."

This difference of opinion persisted for many years, particularly in the area of cardiac surgery where the turf battles were especially hard fought.

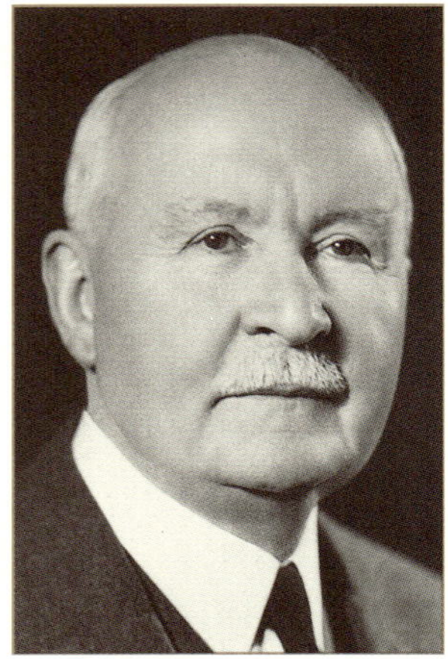

Carl Eggers, M.D.
Chairman

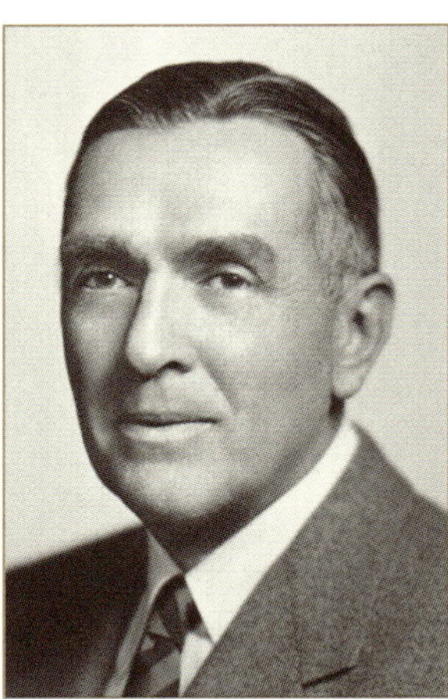

Cameron Haight, M.D.
Vice-Chairman

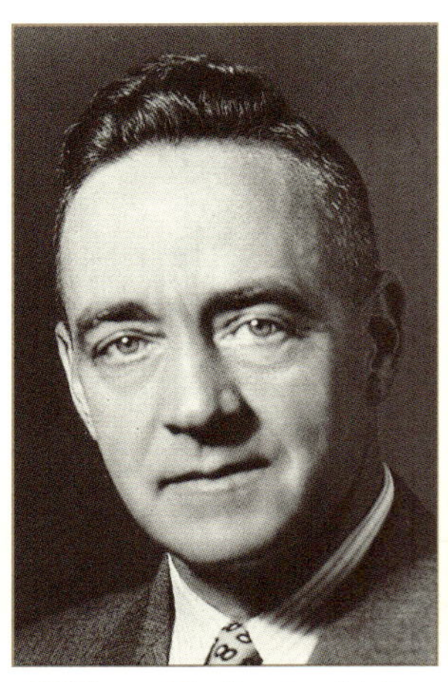

William M. Tuttle, M.D.
Secretary-Treasurer

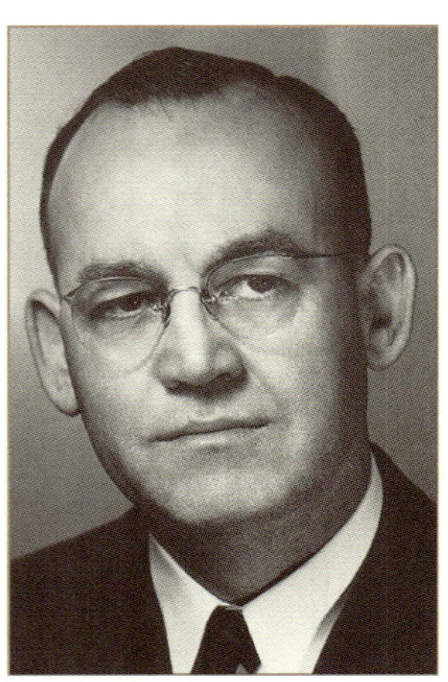

William Adams, M.D.

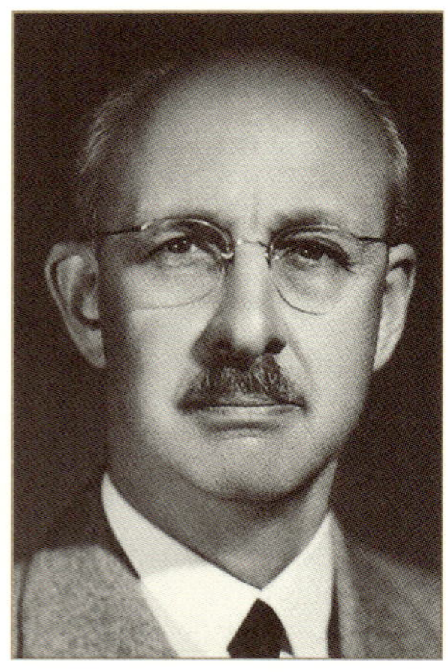

Emile Holman, M.D.

The early work in cardiac surgery was accomplished by men such as Alfred Blalock and Robert Gross, who considered themselves to be general surgeons. Evarts Graham felt he was a general surgeon with a special interest in the chest. Only later was cardiac surgery considered to be a part of thoracic surgery.

THE ORGANIZATIONAL MEETING

Despite problems, the formation of the Board proceeded and the organizational meeting was held in Detroit, Michigan, on October 2, 1948. The original Board members were:

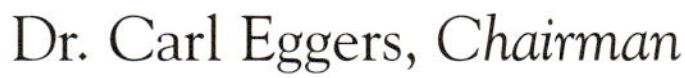

Dr. Carl Eggers, *Chairman*
Dr. Cameron Haight, *Vice-Chairman*
Dr. William M. Tuttle, *Secretary-Treasurer*
Dr. William Adams
Dr. Frank Berry
Dr. Brian Blades
Dr. Thomas Burford
Dr. Michael DeBakey
Dr. Emile Holman
Dr. George Humphreys
Dr. Richard Sweet

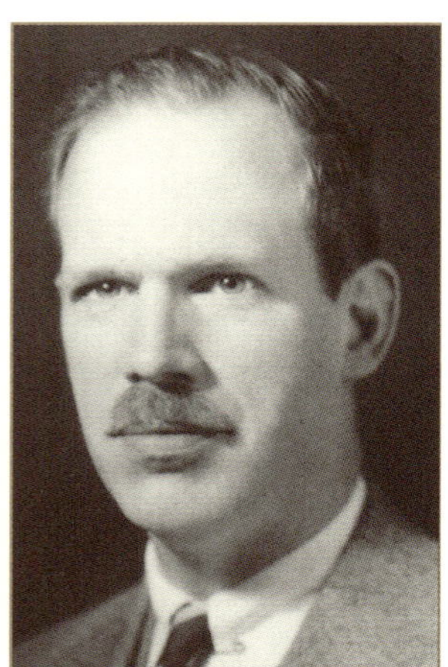

George Humphreys, M.D.

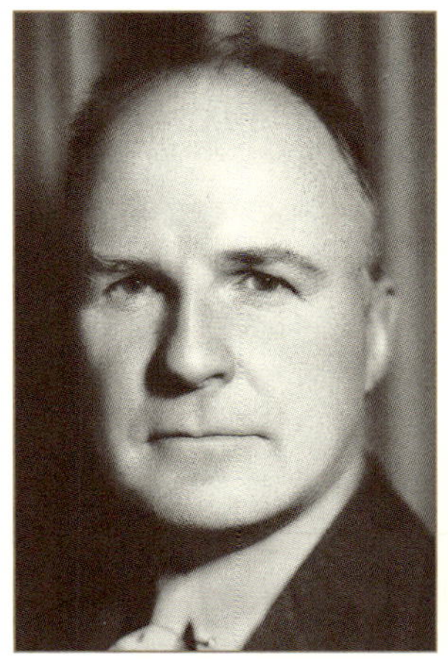
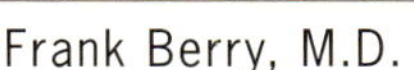
Frank Berry, M.D.

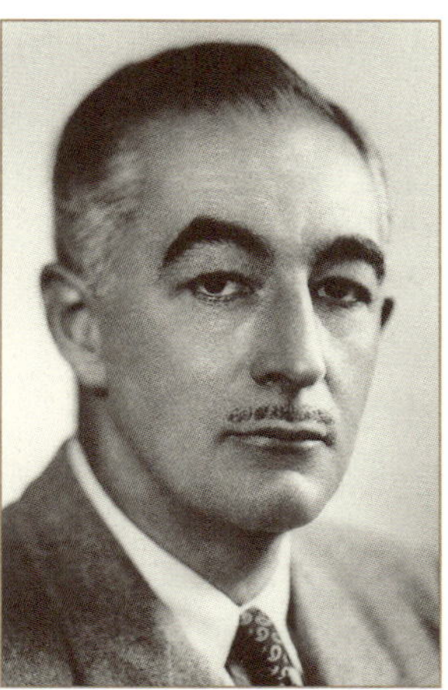
Brian Blades, M.D.

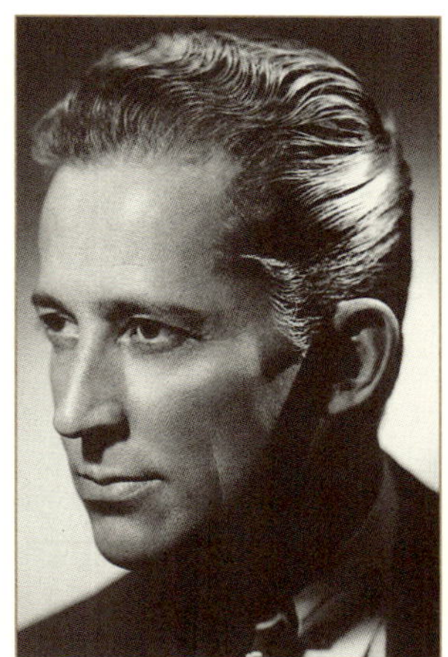
Thomas Burford, M.D.

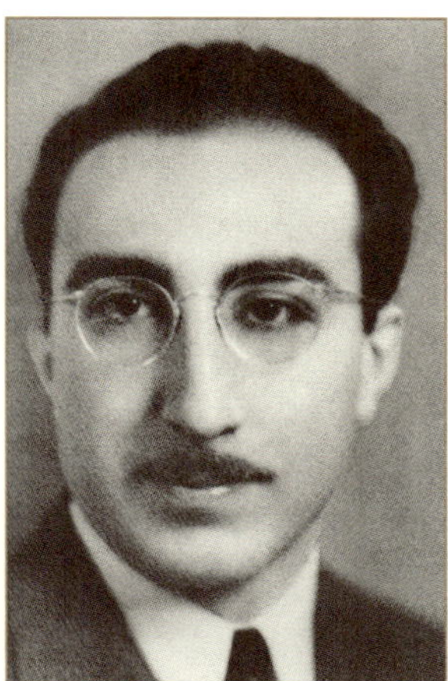
Michael DeBakey, M.D.

At about this same time, Mrs. Louise Sper had her first contact with the Board. She had worked previously as a secretary for a group of thoracic surgeons in Detroit headed by Dr. E. J. O'Brien. Dr. Tuttle was a member of this group from which Louise had resigned in late 1946 when her son, Leslie, was born. When Dr. Tuttle was elected Secretary-Treasurer of the Board, he asked Louise to be responsible for the correspondence and record-keeping of the Board. At that time it was believed the position would require one and one-half days a week. Since there was no office at the time, work was done in Louise's kitchen. Files were kept in a cardboard box. Dr. Tuttle is said to have held Leslie on his lap not infrequently to keep him quiet during these sessions.

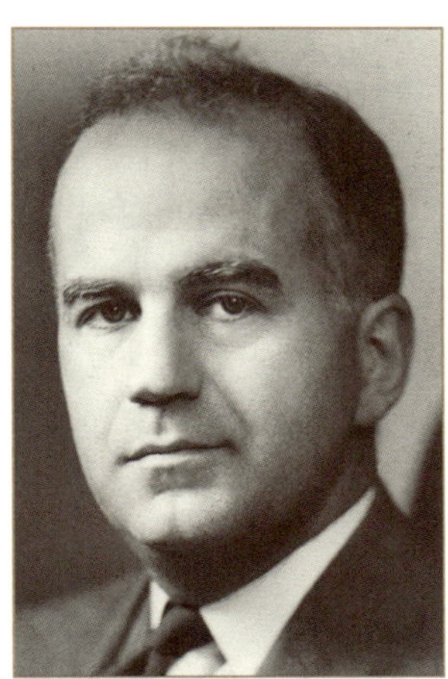
Richard Sweet, M.D.

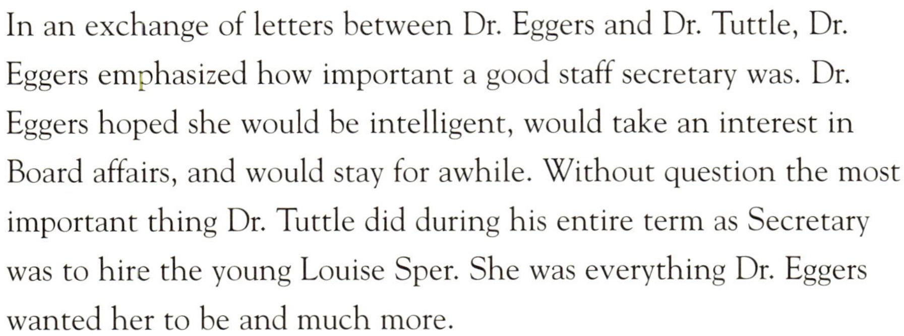
In an exchange of letters between Dr. Eggers and Dr. Tuttle, Dr. Eggers emphasized how important a good staff secretary was. Dr. Eggers hoped she would be intelligent, would take an interest in Board affairs, and would stay for awhile. Without question the most important thing Dr. Tuttle did during his entire term as Secretary was to hire the young Louise Sper. She was everything Dr. Eggers wanted her to be and much more.

IT HAS BEEN SUGGESTED THAT THE CHOICE OF THE FIRST BOARD MEMBERS WAS GREATLY INFLUENCED—IF NOT DICTATED BY—THE PIONEERING GIANTS OF THE ASSOCIATION. THE VARYING PHILOSOPHIES OF THESE MASTER SURGEONS WERE REFLECTED IN THEIR DISCIPLES.

EARLY ACTIVITIES AND DIRECTIONS

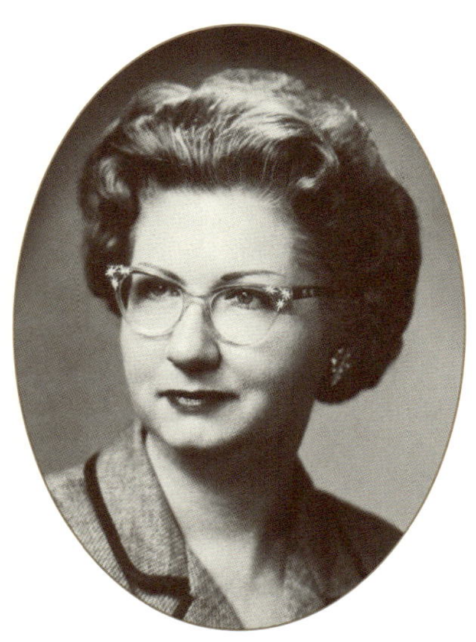

The young Louise Sper.

In January 1949 the office of the Board was established at the Herman Kiefer Hospital in Detroit where it remained until August 1970. The Board borrowed one thousand dollars from the American Association for Thoracic Surgery to get started. Dr. Tuttle managed to obtain furniture at a discount from a patient.

One can speculate that organization of the Board was stimulated by a competing proposal from the American College of Chest Physicians to establish an American Board of Diseases of the Chest.

Some of the reasons for the decisions made are still a mystery. Why was the Board not named the American Board of Thoracic Surgery when this had been suggested by a number of physicians involved in the process and had appeared in some of the preliminary correspondence? The reason was never clearly stated in the records but probably had something to do with the close relationship between the American Board of Surgery and the Board of Thoracic Surgery. It was originally intended that the American Board of Surgery would be responsible for all actions of the Board of Thoracic Surgery and that the Board of Thoracic Surgery would be subsidiary to the American Board of Surgery. However, when attorneys pointed out that this meant responsibility for the debts of the Board of Thoracic Surgery, the Board was quickly made an affiliate with independent functioning.

THE FIRST MEMBERS OF THE BOARD CARRIED A GREAT RESPONSIBILITY AND, DESPITE THEIR DIFFERENT BACKGROUNDS AND PERSONALITIES, THEY WERE DEVOTED TO THE BOARD.

A rotating term of membership by a stagger system was put in place but was not instituted for several of the early years of the Board. The term of membership was originally five years but was changed to six years in 1961. It has been suggested that the choice of the first Board members was greatly influenced—if not dictated by—the pioneering giants of the Association: Churchill, Lambert, O'Brien, Graham, Alexander, Ochsner, and others. The varying philosophies of these master surgeons were reflected in their disciples.

Unity and Factions

It is important to talk about the first members of the Board. They carried a great responsibility and, despite their different backgrounds and personalities, they were devoted to the Board. All of them put forth great effort to make the new Board a success. George Humphreys,[1] one of the last remaining members of the original Board, has described the background of the Board and its members in a fascinating article. He notes that there were two main groups: The master general surgeons were dominant and believed that thoracic surgery should not be a separate specialty. They thought that any well-trained surgeon with a good anesthetist should be able to include thoracic surgery among his or her skills. (Note that Dr. Humphreys used the word *her*. Few of the Founders anticipated that women would become the force in thoracic surgery that they have. Nonetheless, some foresighted individuals saw that the sea changes in thoracic surgery would include the gender profile of surgeons among many other things.)

[1] Humphreys, G. Origins of the American Board of Thoracic Surgery. *Ann Thorac Surg*, 1985; 39:290–291.

TECHNICAL ADVANCES WERE MANY, AND ANTIBIOTICS HAD HAD A TREMENDOUS IMPACT ON INFECTION. WORLD WAR II HAD PROVIDED A MAJOR STIMULUS THAT GAVE MANY YOUNG SURGEONS CONCENTRATED EXPERIENCE IN TREATING THORACIC TRAUMA.

Drs. Adams, Berry, DeBakey, Eggers, Holman, Humphreys, and Sweet were primarily general surgeons doing thoracic surgery. Drs. Blades, Burford, Haight, and Tuttle all considered thoracic surgery to be a specialty in its own right.

No one in his right mind, it was thought, could make a living at thoracic surgery. However, by 1948 the situation was changing rapidly. Technical advances were many, and antibiotics had had a tremendous impact on infection. World War II had provided a major stimulus that gave many young surgeons concentrated experience in treating thoracic trauma. Successful surgical treatment for congenital cardiovascular anomalies had also made its start. The older generation finally recognized that certification in thoracic surgery could no longer be denied.

MAJOR PERSONALITIES

Carl Eggers was the natural choice for Chairman. He had been in the forefront of every discussion of certification and had chaired every committee in which the subject had been considered. Herbert Maier, who was so closely associated with Dr. Eggers, described him as having a profound interest in the training of young surgeons. Dr. Maier admired Dr. Eggers' commitment to the formation of a thoracic board. He noted in later recollections that Dr. Eggers was keenly interested in postgraduate medical education and was also a strong advocate of thorough training in general surgery before branching into a surgical specialty. He had been chairman of such a

"THE PRESIDENT OF THE AMERICAN ASSOCIATION OF THORACIC SURGERY HAS JUST APPOINTED A COMMITTEE TO CONFER WITH THE SPECIAL COMMITTEE OF THE AMERICAN SURGICAL ASSOCIATION... TO COMPLETE ARRANGEMENTS FOR THE FORMATION OF THE BOARD OF THORACIC SURGERY..."

TELEPHONE, BUTTERFIELD 8-5753

CARL EGGERS, M.D.
850 PARK AVENUE
NEW YORK 21, N.Y.

July 11th,1947.

JUL 12 1947

Dr. J. Stewart Rodman,
Secretary, The American Board of Surgery,
225 South Fifteenth Street,
Philadelphia 2, Penna.

My dear Doctor Rodman:-

The President of the American Association of Thoracic Surgery has just appointed a Committee to confer with the special Committee of the American Surgical Association in order to complete the arrangements for the formation of the Board of Thoracic Surgery. The Committee consists of

Dr. I. A. Bigger.
Dr. Brian Blades.
Dr. Cameron Haight.
Dr. Richard H. Meade Jr.
Dr. Carl Eggers, Chairman.

I suppose the membership of the Committee of the American Surgical Association remains unchanged. I shall therefore make contact with Dr. Nathan Womack, its Chairman, and give you a copy of any communication I may send him.

With best regards.

Sincerely yours,
Carl Eggers
Carl Eggers, M. D.

CE/LS

Dr. Eggers' letter to J. Stewart Rodman, Secretary of the American Board of Surgery, proposing formation of a Board of Thoracic Surgery.

THE EXTRAORDINARY CORRESPONDENCE DR. EGGERS CARRIED ON AT THIS TIME, PARTICULARLY WITH DR. TUTTLE, IS A REMARKABLE DEMONSTRATION OF HIS ORGANIZATIONAL ABILITY AND DEVOTION TO THE BOARD.

committee at the New York Academy of Medicine and "gave great attention to any committee assignments that he might have."

George Humphreys recalled the benign control he exerted over a group of very opinionated "boys," control characterized by Teutonic discipline but softened by the tolerance of age. Dr. Tuttle thought that Dr. Eggers looked like Santa Claus. The extraordinary correspondence Dr. Eggers carried on at this time, particularly with Dr. Tuttle, is a remarkable demonstration of his organizational ability and devotion to the Board.

Cameron Haight, who was elected Vice-Chairman of the Board, brought much of Dr. Alexander's philosophy of thoracic surgery to the Board. He followed Dr. Eggers as Chairman, when Dr. Eggers stepped down in 1952.

Secretary-Treasurer William Tuttle remained in that position until his death in 1962. More than any other Board member, he represented the young thoracic surgeons, particularly those who had served in the Armed Forces. Dr. Tuttle was a stormy petrel, but he provided energetic leadership as Secretary during the early years of the Board.

Thomas Burford, easily the most handsome member of the group, was a strong advocate of thoracic surgery as a separate specialty and insisted that general surgeons had no business doing occasional chest operations. Frank Berry, on the other hand, was firm in his conviction that thoracic surgery was an extension of general surgery.

THESE MEN HAD STRONG PERSONALITIES AND WERE ACCUSTOMED TO EXERCISING CONSIDERABLE AUTHORITY IN THEIR OWN WORLDS.

Emile Holman was the only man on the Board who had the distinction of having been trained by Halsted. He was a courtly, erudite gentleman for whom all the Board members had enormous respect. Brian Blades, another believer in thoracic surgery as an extension of general surgery, made important contributions to the Association as editor of its journal.

George Humphreys considered himself as a *self-taught* thoracic surgeon and was one of the early entrants into the emerging field of cardiac surgery. Richard Sweet, a superb surgeon and scholar, contributed much to the surgery of the esophagus and mediastinum. He followed Dr. Haight as Chairman of the Board but remained in that position for just one year.

Michael DeBakey was a special case. He was the youngest of the Board members but was already very experienced in operating within a committee structure. His decisive presence was invaluable. He did not serve out his term but rather resigned to join the American Board of Surgery.

The final member of the original Board was William Adams who leaned toward the philosophy of restrictive specialization. He was a quiet, gentle, extremely capable person who made things work. Dr. Adams followed Dr. Sweet as Chairman and was one of the last original members to retire from the Board in 1957.

"THE BOARD OF THORACIC SURGERY WAS FORMED BY THE ASSOCIATION UNDER THE AMERICAN BOARD OF SURGERY... THIS BOARD HAS BEEN SET UP WITH THE IDEA OF SPONSORING THE HIGHEST QUALIFICATIONS IN THORACIC SURGERY..."

To emphasize just what leaders these men were, nine of the original eleven members served as President of the American Association for Thoracic Surgery at some point in their careers. These men had strong personalities and were accustomed to exercising considerable authority in their own worlds. Inevitably, clashes occurred, principally over the relationship of thoracic surgery to general surgery. Despite these clashes, the members were all imbued with the idea of strengthening the specialty of thoracic surgery and were devoted to the future of the Board.

The Founder Members

Dr. Eggers was given the first certificate and the other Founder members received their certificates in the order of their election to membership in the Association. One notable exception was Dr. Churchill, who received certificate No. 174 instead of No. 13, to which he was entitled, because he had delayed so long in applying. This, of course, reflected Dr. Churchill's attitude toward thoracic surgery as a specialty. Dr. Evarts A. Graham also had a high-numbered certificate, even though he held Certificate No. 1 for his American Board of Surgery certification.

As the Board members attempted to complete the list of Founder Members, an additional group of candidates was agreed upon after consultation with the American Board of Surgery. These were surgeons who were neither members of the American Association for Thoracic Surgery nor diplomates of the American Board of Surgery.

DR. EGGERS WAS GIVEN THE FIRST CERTIFICATE AND THE OTHER FOUNDER MEMBERS RECEIVED THEIR CERTIFICATES IN THE ORDER OF THEIR ELECTION TO MEMBERSHIP IN THE ASSOCIATION.

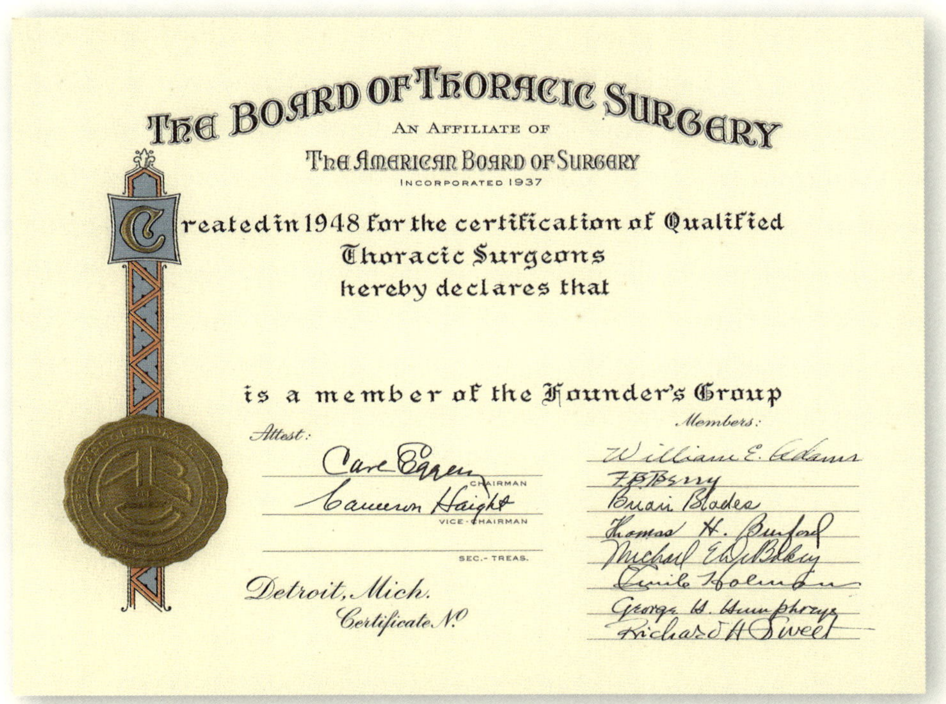
The Board of Thoracic Surgery
An Affiliate of
The American Board of Surgery
Incorporated 1937
Created in 1948 for the certification of Qualified Thoracic Surgeons
hereby declares that

is a member of the Founder's Group

Attest:
Carl Eggers — Chairman
Cameron Haight — Vice-Chairman
Sec.-Treas.

Detroit, Mich.
Certificate No.

Members:
William E. Adams
F B Berry
Brian Blades
Thomas H. Burford
Michael E. DeBakey
Emile Holman
George H. Humphreys
Richard H Sweet

First Board certificate.

Their training, because of the period in which it was taken, did not qualify them to become certified by the American Board of Surgery. However, upon careful scrutiny by the Board of Thoracic Surgery and adequate evidence of proficiency, they became eligible for consideration as Founder Members.

In 1951 the Founders group was closed, a year later than originally planned. Two hundred twenty-eight surgeons were selected for the Founders group and were sent their certificates. Another name was officially added to the Founders Group many years later. Dr. Huang

1949 An informational booklet about the Board is published.

1951 The Founders group is closed, with two hundred twenty-eight surgeons selected for membership.

THE BOARD
OF
THORACIC SURGERY
AN AFFILIATE OF THE
AMERICAN BOARD OF SURGERY, INC.

BOOKLET
OF INFORMATION
1949

OFFICE OF THE SECRETARY
DR. WM. M. TUTTLE
1151 Taylor Avenue
Detroit 2, Michigan

First Board information booklet.

Chia-ssu, who had trained in Ann Arbor and who later had been President of the Chinese Academy of Medical Sciences, was made a Founder member, but this honor was withdrawn by the Board when it was thought that he had supported China during the Korean war. In 1979 he visited the United States. Shortly after that his original certificate was found in the Board office, and it was felt to be appropriate to award it to him. It was delivered to him in China, with appropriate ceremony, by Dr. Myron Wegman, Dean of the University of Michigan School of Public Health, who was visiting China at that time.

FIRST PUBLICATION

In 1949 a booklet of information was published (*left*). It contained necessary details regarding the Board as well as the requirements for certification. There was a section on training requirements, which in an early draft had contained a reference to endoscopy, but this was removed before publication.

While all this was going on, a letter was received from a surgeon in Chicago stating that "The American Board of Thoracic Surgery" had been incorporated by five Chicago surgeons on December 22, 1948, in Washington, D.C. None was certified by the American Board of Surgery nor was any of them a member of the Association. It was suggested that the Board of Thoracic Surgery could not function so long as the other Board was incorporated. Dr. Tuttle answered the letter in his own inimitable way, and the group, whatever its intentions,

"WE HAVE LEARNED A GREAT DEAL. WE MUST NEVER FORGET THAT WE HAVE RESPONSIBILITY TOWARDS THE PUBLIC. THEREFORE, WE HAVE TO SEE THAT WE RECOMMEND FOR CERTIFICATION BY THE BOARD, ABLE MEN OF GOOD CHARACTER...."

disappeared from view. The documents later found their way to the Board offices. Among other things, Dr. Tuttle stated, "I have recently received your letter of January 7, 1949, in which you mention the granting of a charter from Washington to form apparently a second Board of Thoracic Surgery. As far as I know, socialized medicine is not in effect, and I do not know what power Washington has to form any certification board in surgery.

"The Board of Thoracic Surgery was formed by the Association under the American Board of Surgery...This Board has been set up with the idea of sponsoring the highest qualifications in thoracic surgery. There are a number of individuals who may not be qualified for this Board, and if they are not, then they will have to resort undoubtedly to spurious boards. There is, however, only one Board of Thoracic Surgery, and it is on this letterhead that this letter is being written you.

"...You are eligible to apply for the Founders' Group without examination, and I am herewith enclosing an application blank."

To the best of my knowledge, no one of these individuals ever applied for the Founders Group of the Board of Thoracic Surgery.

The Board completed its infancy in 1952 when Dr. Eggers stepped down as Chairman. In one of his last letters to Dr. Tuttle he emphasized the Board's responsibility to the public. He stated, "We have learned a great deal. We must never forget that we have responsibility

1951 Founder member group closes.

1952 Stagger system of rotation of Board members begins. First Chairman, Dr. Carl Eggers, retires.

towards the public. Therefore, we have to see that we recommend for certification by the Board, able men of good character. Still, we should not become hard boiled. We also have a responsibility towards the men who have prepared themselves for the practice of thoracic surgery."

This was typical of the man who had done so much for the Board and thoracic surgery. On his retirement the other Board members presented him with a gold watch.

CHAPTER 3

The Early Years

1949 The first written examination is given August 1; the first oral examination is administered October 15, 1949.

1950 The Board is granted a corporate charter by the State of Michigan. The original bylaws are readopted.

1954 First discussion of cardiac surgery as part of thoracic surgery. No credit for preceptor training.

THE FIRST EXAMINATIONS

At the same time the Board was dealing with the selection of Founder Members, they began to administer the first examinations. The first written examination was given on August 1, 1949. Twenty-eight candidates took this examination, and there were six failures. This essay examination contained questions that addressed anatomy, pathology, physiology, and surgical technique. Most interesting, in the light of subsequent events, was the inclusion of a question on cardiac surgery. The written examination contained questions in two parts (*page* 46). Five of the six questions in each part were to be answered.

The first oral examination was administered in Chicago on October 15, 1949. It was given to 20 candidates. Of these, 15 passed and were issued certificates. From the beginning, prominent and promising thoracic surgeons were selected to help administer the oral examinations. This was often a testing ground for future Board membership.

The examination process was not without its problems both for examiners and examinees. Dr. Berry was very upset about the handling of the written examination booklets. In a letter he wanted to know: "What the hell do you want me to do with the damn books?"

1955 First representative to ABS Examination Committee is appointed.

1956 Examination is broadened to include more questions in cardiovascular surgery.

Questions from the first Board examination.

QUESTIONS FROM THE FIRST BOARD EXAMINATION

Part One

1. What technical improvements do you consider to be the most important in extending the scope of thoracic surgery during the past 30 years, and why?
2. Discuss the alterations in physiology which occur in children with congenital heart anomalies resulting in cyanosis.
3. Describe in detail the essential surgical anatomy of the left upper pulmonary lobe.
4. Discuss the indications for the use of streptomycin in thoracic surgery. Include dosage and method of administration and length of treatment in the various conditions in which you would use it.
5. Discuss the pathology of cystic disease of the lung.
6. Describe the alterations in cardiorespiratory physiology resulting from:
   a. Large *flail* segment of chest wall
   b. An open chest wound two centimeters in diameter.
   c. A large pulmonary laceration with closed chest wall.

Part Two

1. Discuss the differential diagnosis of lesions of the superior mediastinum.
2. Describe your postoperative management of a sixty year old man following removal of his right lung. What complications do you fear and how would you diagnose and treat each?
3. Discuss the indications for thoracoplasty in the treatment of pulmonary tuberculosis.

1957 Serious differences arise between ABS and BTS on general surgery training necessary to qualify for BTS certification.

1958 Recorder first used.

1959 First formal representative is appointed to ABS.

$ 1,000 October 2 19 48
Five years after date we promise to pay to
the order of The American Association for Thoracic Surgery
One Thousand and no/100 ---------- Dollars
at
Value received with interest at the rate of 0 per cent per annum.
No. Due October 2, 1953
Carl Eggers, M.D., Chrmn, Board of Thor. Sur
William Tuttle, M.D., Sec'y-Treas.

One thousand dollar promissory note for loan from American Association for Thoracic Surgery.

The books had been sent to Examination Committee members to grade and were to be passed from one member to another. Evidently problems with the schedule of that plan arose to annoy Dr. Berry.

At the second written examination, given early in 1950, one examinee, a self-described "country boy," Herbert Sloan, got lost on his way to the examination site in Detroit where, for the first time he encountered Louise Sper. The second candidate scheduled to take the exam in Detroit that day never did appear.

During his oral examination Gordon Scannell had the temerity to point out to his examiner, whom he knew well, that he was attempting to smoke a filter tip cigarette from the wrong end. According to Dr. Scannell, things went steadily downhill from that point. It must be remembered, however, that at that time the differences between examiner and examinee were not as great as they were later.

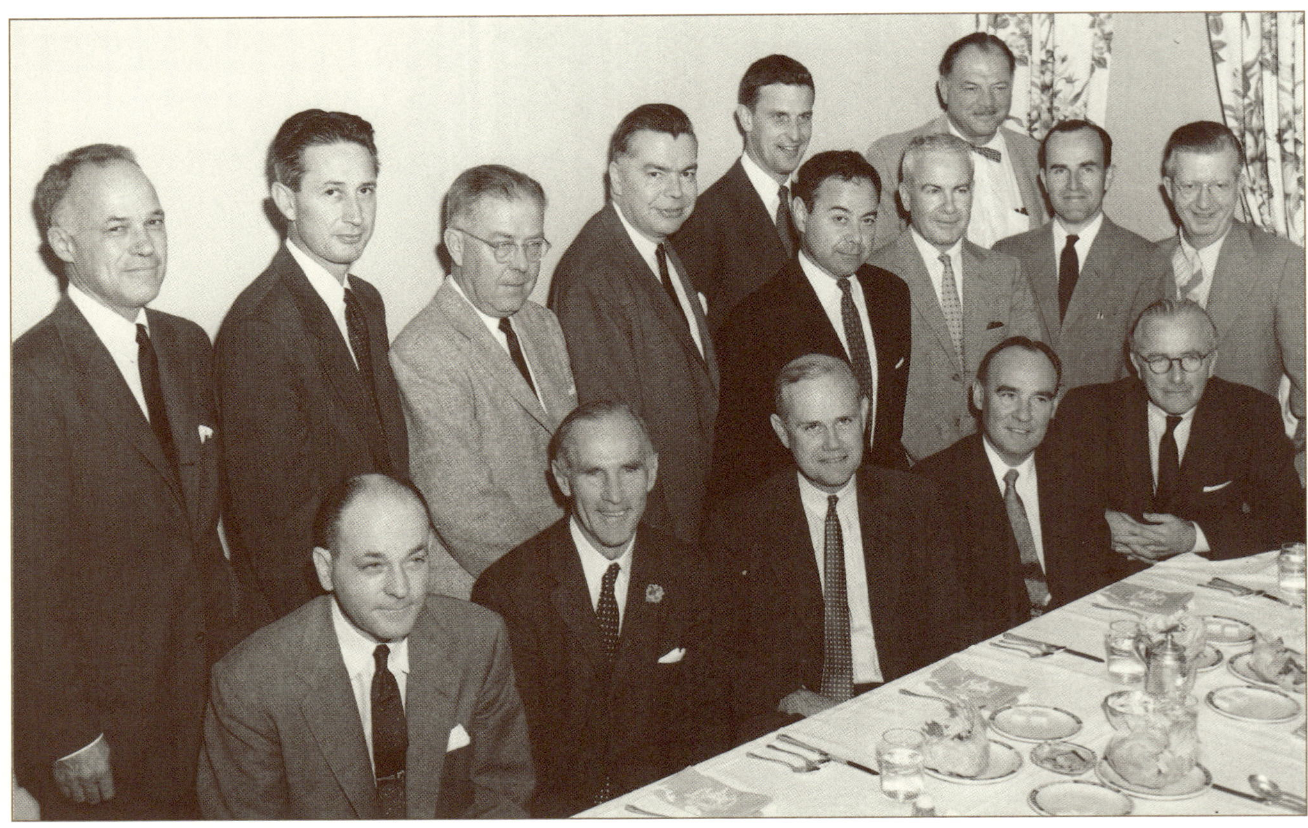

Meeting in San Francisco of Board members and other interested thoracic surgeons (ca. 1956).
Seated, left to right: Dr. Hiram Langston, Dr. Brody Stephens, Dr. Julian Johnson, Dr. John C. Jones, Dr. Lyman A. Brewer.
Standing, left to right: Dr. Robert Wylie, Dr. Orville Grimes, Dr. Joseph Gale, Dr. Herbert Maier, Dr. Benson B. Roe, Dr. Isadore Cohn, Dr. O. Theron Clagett, Dr. Paul Samson, Dr. David Dugan, Dr. Edward Kent.

THE BOARD LOOKS AT TRAINING PROGRAMS

In its first deliberations the Board felt they should not be involved in approving hospitals for the training of thoracic surgeons. The difficulty of serving both as a certifying body for candidates and as the approval mechanism for training programs was noted.

However, it soon became obvious that the candidates and the training programs were part of the same continuum. Thus, a committee was appointed to investigate the issue of program approval in 1949.

A list of provisionally approved residencies was sent to the Council on Medical Education and Hospitals of the American Medical Association in October 1950. Arrangements were made to begin inspection of these hospitals by representatives from the Council.

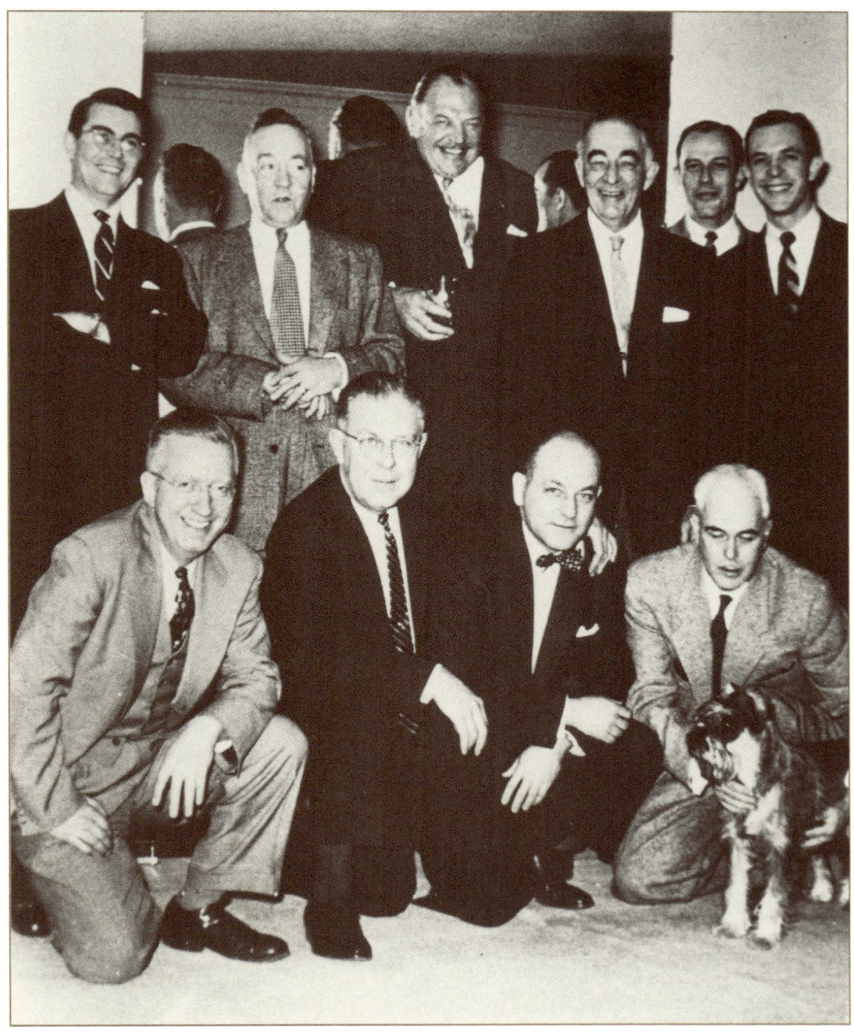

Early meeting of Board members and others in Washington, D.C. at the home of Dr. Brian Blades around 1957.

Bottom row, left to right:
Dr. Edward Kent, Dr. Joseph Gale, Dr. Hiram Langston, Dr. Kennedy, Dr. Blades' dog.

Top row, left to right:
Dr. Paul Adkins, Dr. Bill Tuttle, Dr. Paul "Buck" Samson, Dr. Brian Blades, Dr. Owen Gwathmey, Dr. George Magovern.

EARLY ACTIVITIES

In 1948 the fee for Founder Members had been raised from $25 to $50 and the examination fee to $100, because the Board had already anticipated financial problems. The $1000 the Board had borrowed from the Association in 1948 was repaid in 1949 (*see page* 47).

The original Board members quickly realized that the Board would continue to exist long after they had departed. Thus the custom of obtaining a photograph of each member as he came on the Board was established.

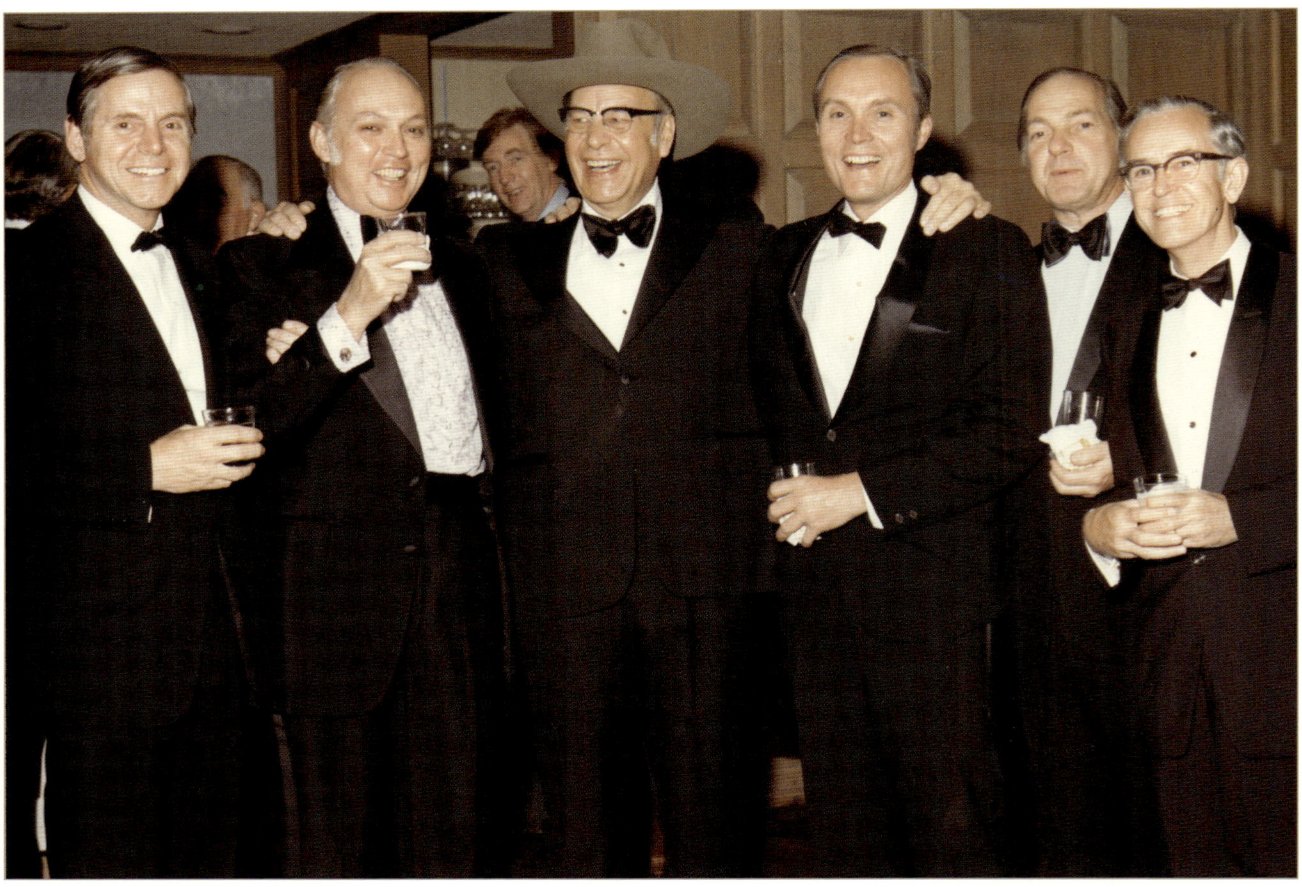

Gathering of former Board members at Emeritus Dinner, Dallas, 1973.
Left to right:
Dr. F. Henry "Bunky" Ellis, Dr. Myron Wheat. Dr. Don Paulson, Dr. James Malm, Dr. Jay Ankeney, Dr. Robert Ellison.

As the Board matured, several pleasant habit patterns developed. One was the practice of eating dinner together the evening before a Board meeting. These dinners increased the camaraderie and good fellowship, which became extremely important in the harmonious functioning of the Board. One especially rewarding custom was to have the label removed from one of the wine bottles and, after it had dried, each person signed the label, often with a message. Louise Sper collected and saved these over the years (*see page 51*). They tell a fascinating history of the many wonderful experiences the ever-changing Board members enjoyed. Commenting on some photographs made during such events, Dr. Tuttle noted the frequent appearance of the "flexed arm syndrome."

THE BOARD OF THORACIC SURGERY THEN DECIDED TO EXAMINE CANDIDATES IN CARDIOVASCULAR SURGERY AND TO ASSUME RESPONSIBILITY FOR INCLUDING CARDIOVASCULAR SURGERY IN THE FIELD OF THORACIC SURGERY.

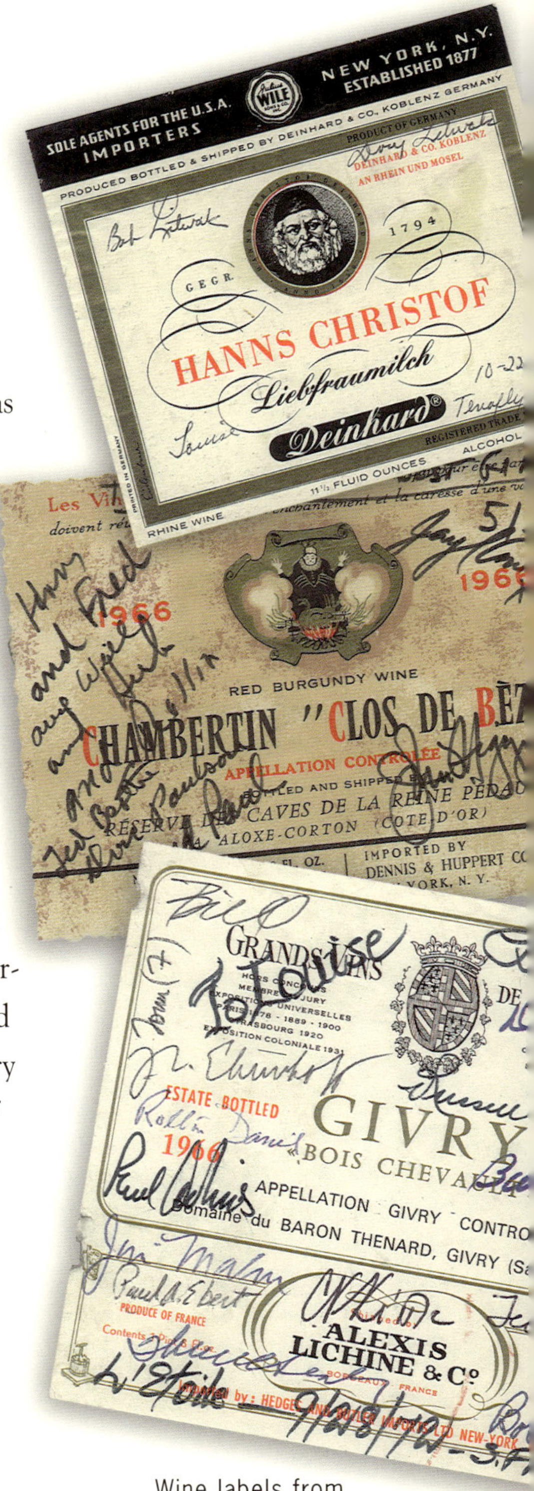

Wine labels from Louise Sper's collection.

Another important Board function was the emeritus dinner, which was held approximately every five years. To this were invited all present and past Board members together with their wives or friends. These black tie affairs were always held in an outstanding restaurant in a major city and allowed previous Board members to renew old friendships and learn about the present status of the Board (*pages 52–54*).

THE MATURATION PROCESS

In 1950 the Board was granted a corporate charter by the state of Michigan. The original bylaws were readopted.

As additional examinations were given, concern was expressed about the candidates' weaknesses in the history of thoracic surgery, the interpretation of x-rays, and tuberculosis. The original Board members had worked together for five years. It was felt this continuity was necessary during the Board's first years, but by 1957 all the original members of the Board had been replaced with the exception of Dr. Tuttle, who remained as Secretary.

INTEREST IN CARDIOVASCULAR SURGERY RISES

It was during these years that the question of cardiovascular surgery first surfaced. In the evaluation of training programs it was noted that the number of cases of pulmonary tuberculosis was decreasing, whereas the number of cardiovascular cases was increasing. Other groups began to discuss the desirability of establishing a certifying

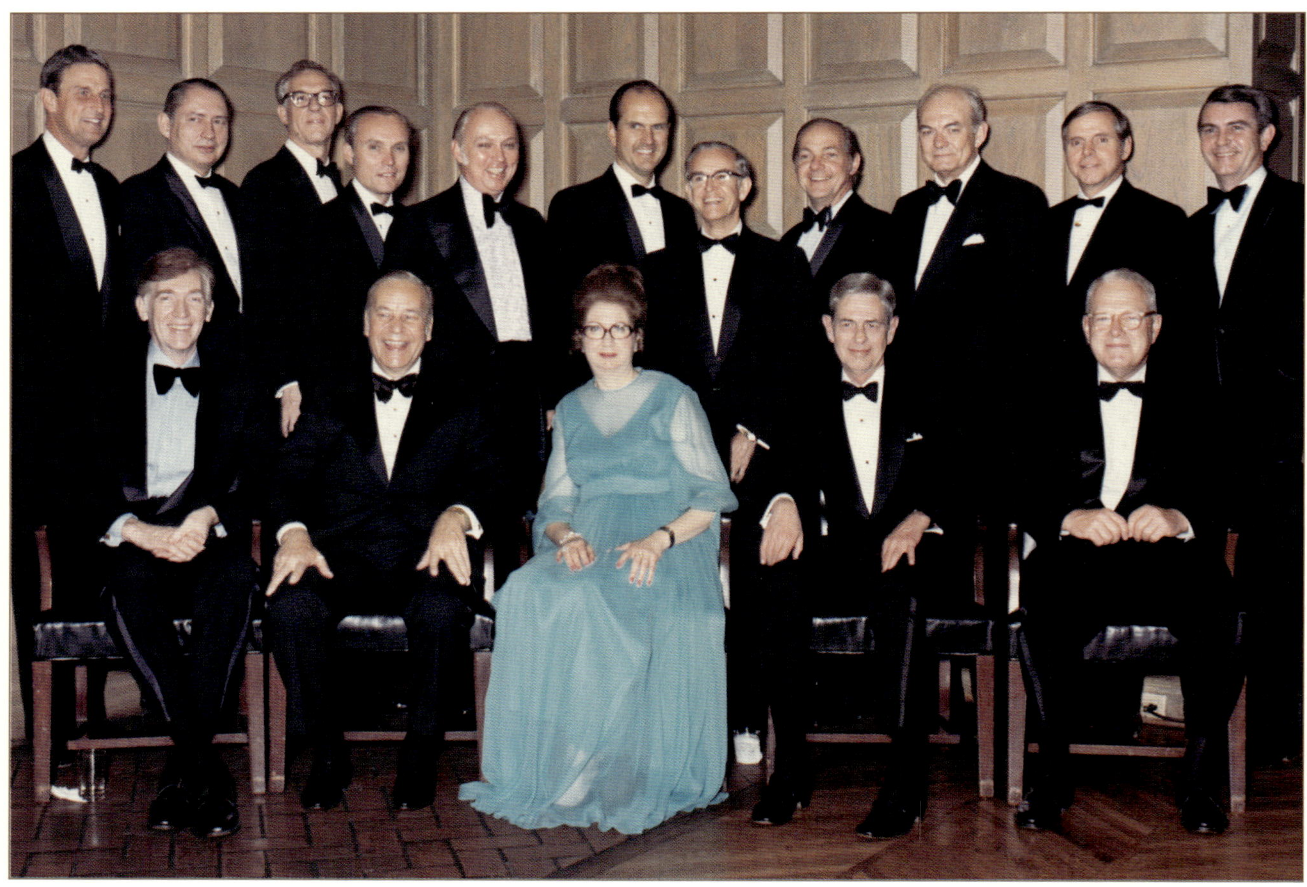

Dallas, 1973.
Seated, left to right: Dr. Fred Kittle, Dr. Don Paulson, Louise Sper, Dr. Rollin Daniel, Dr. Herbert Sloan.
Standing, left to right: Dr. Ben Roe, Dr. Ralph Alley, Dr. Tom Ferguson, Dr. James Malm, Dr. Myron Wheat, Dr. Russell Nelson, Dr. Robert Ellison, Dr. Jay Ankeney, Dr. Will Sealy, Dr. F. Henry Ellis, Dr. Paul Adkins.

Board for cardiovascular surgery. A questionnaire to directors of thoracic training programs showed that most programs included cardiovascular surgery, but the residents performed very little of it.

As the discussion continued, it was determined that no other group wished to assume responsibility for establishing a separate Board of Cardiovascular Surgery. The Board of Thoracic Surgery then decided to examine candidates in cardiovascular surgery and to assume responsibility for including cardiovascular surgery in the field of thoracic surgery. Still, the Board members did not wish to issue a special certificate for cardiovascular surgery. It was simply to be a part of thoracic surgery.

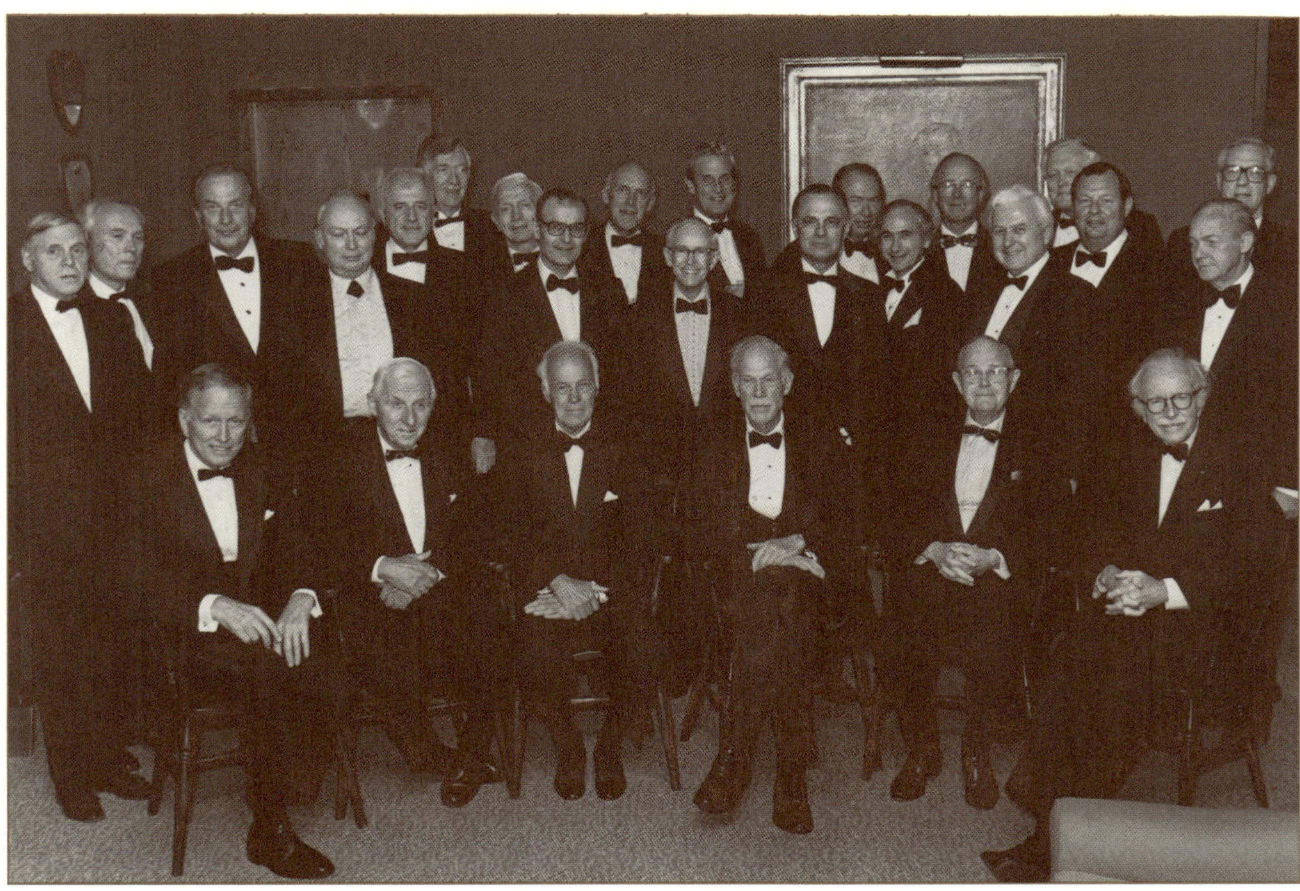

1977 Princeton Club, New York City.
Seated left to right: Dr. Denton Cooley, Dr. Gordon Scannell, Dr. Robert Wylie, Dr. George Humphreys, Dr. William Adams, Dr. Lyman Brewer.
Standing, left to right: Dr. F. Henry Ellis, Dr. James Malm, Dr. Donald Effler, Dr. Myron Wheat, Dr. Hans Ehrenhaft, Dr. Fred Kittle, Dr. Henry Bahnson, Dr. Watts Webb, Dr. James Maloney, Dr. Robert Ellison, Dr. Ben Roe, Dr. Frank Spencer, Dr. Ralph Alley, Dr. Albert Starr, Dr. Sterling Edwards, Dr. Edward Beattie, Dr. Philip Bernatz, Dr. Hal Urschel, Dr. Jay Ankeney, Dr. Tom Ferguson.

At this same time the question arose regarding the desirability of changing the name of the Board. This discussion continued for several years before the name was finally changed to The American Board of Thoracic Surgery in 1971.

BOARD ROTATIONS

At the time of his retirement in 1952 Dr. Carl Eggers believed the Board was on solid footing and its future assured.

Cameron Haight, who had followed Dr. Eggers as Chairman, was in turn followed by Richard Sweet and William Adams. Replacing the original members as they retired were: Julian Johnson, Joseph Gale, Paul Samson, John Jones (the first Chairman who was not a member of the original Board), Robert Wylie, Edward Kent, Hiram Langston,

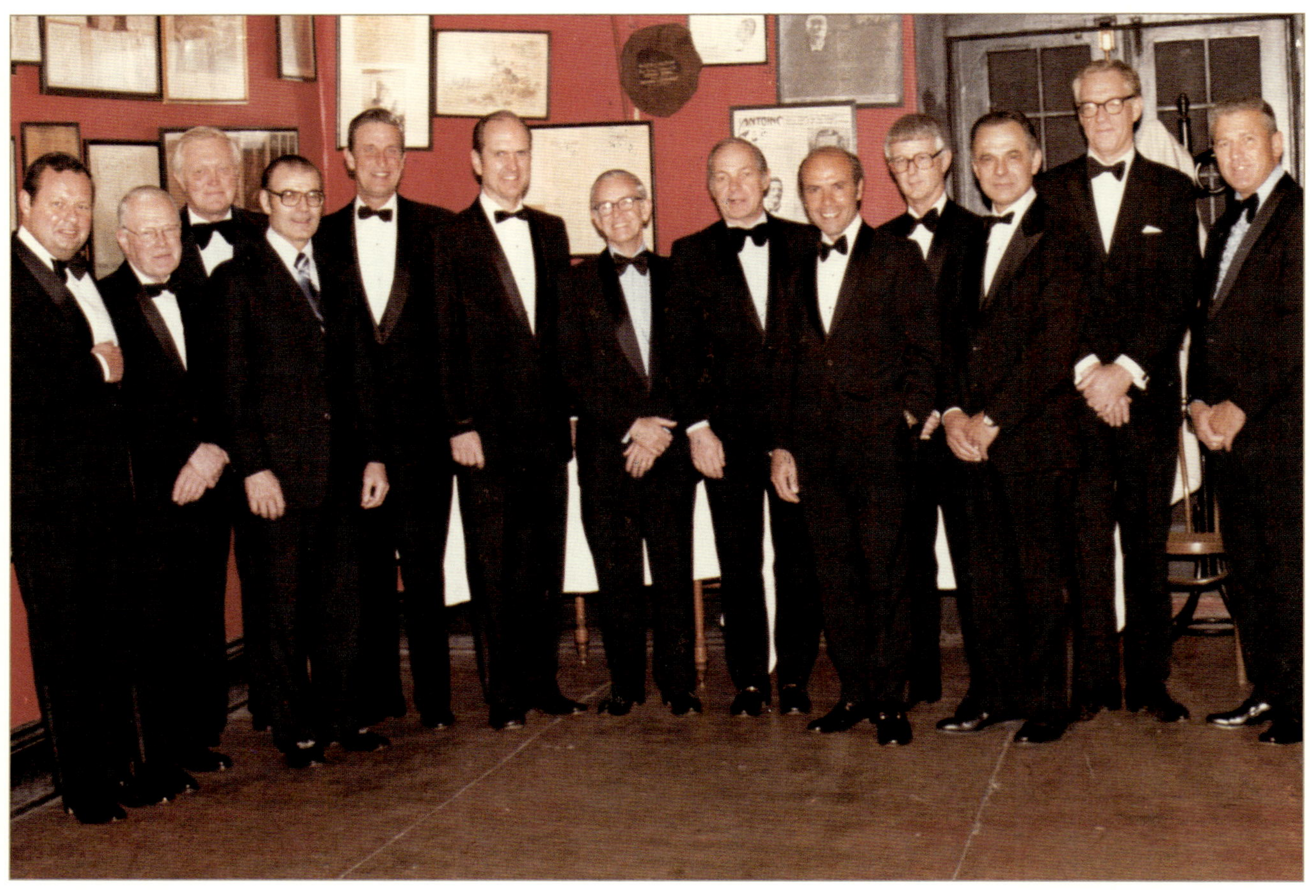

New Orleans, 1978.
Left to right: Dr. Harold Urschel, Dr. Herbert Sloan, Dr. Philip E. Bernatz, Dr. Watts Webb, Dr. Benson B. Roe, Dr. Russell M. Nelson, Dr. Robert G. Ellison, Dr. Jay L. Ankeney, Dr. Hassan Najafi, Dr. John W. Kirklin, Dr. Frank C. Spencer, Dr. Thomas B. Ferguson, Dr. Donald G. Mulder.

O. Theron "Jim" Clagett, Herbert Maier, and Robert Shaw. The other Board members who replaced retiring members were: Anthony Curreri, Henry Bahnson, Lyman Brewer III, John Strieder, Paul Sanger, Rollin Daniel, Francis Byron, and Edward Beattie.

OTHER ISSUES

A statement by Dr. Brian Blades was made in the Journal of Thoracic Surgery in 1953, the essence of which was that the Board had no interest in how its diplomates were compensated. Rather, he said the purpose of the Board was to establish adequate standards of training in thoracic surgery and to conduct examinations to determine the qualifications of the candidates.

CHAPTER 4

The Board Comes of Age

1953 Attention is paid to the problem of program approval and the establishment of a tripartite residency review committee. This trend continues throughout the 1950s and 1960s.

1956 The Board feels that a candidate should be examined in the entire field of thoracic surgery, whatever his experience.

1960–1963 Emphasis on cardiovascular surgery grows. Term on Board increases to six years from five.

THE MACHINERY TURNS

In the late 1950s, the Board members began to concentrate on their major functions. They evaluated the credentials of applicants for examination. They administered the examination. Together with the Council on Medical Education and Hospitals of the American Medical Association, the Board evaluated training programs.

Various administrative concerns arose and were worked out: Louise Sper was given authority to sign checks. A little later an annuity of $100 monthly to begin at age 60 was established for her. She was also bonded for $5000. Louise was esteemed very highly by all members of the Board because she was a conscientious, intelligent worker and because of the depth of her commitment to the organization and its members.

Having each Board member sign each certificate had become increasingly onerous. The certificate was changed so that only the Chairman, Vice-Chairman, and the Secretary signed it. The Board agreed that its members should be reimbursed for travel and living

NEAR THE END OF THE DECADE **[1950s]** THE AMERICAN ASSOCIATION FOR THORACIC SURGERY MADE A DECISION THAT ANY CANDIDATE FOR MEMBERSHIP MUST BE CERTIFIED BY THE BOARD OF THORACIC SURGERY.

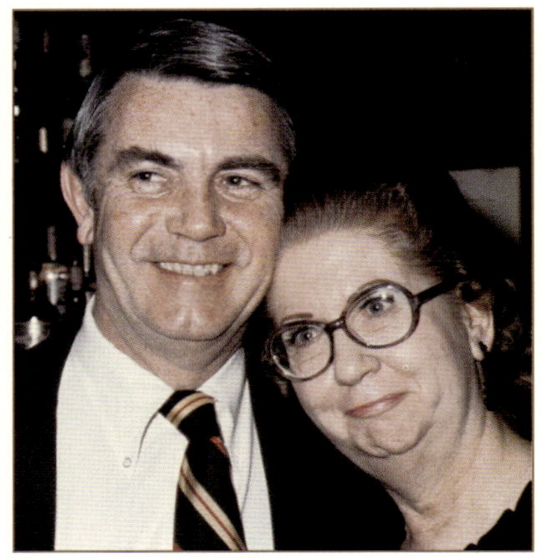

Louise Sper and Dr. Paul Adkins, Board Chairman, 1975–1977.

expenses when they attended Board meetings, whether or not the meetings were held in conjunction with another meeting.

The Credentials Committee evaluated applicants for examination. Questionable applications were brought to the entire Board for discussion. The Board was not always consistent in its deliberations. For example, they had decided that no credit would be given for foreign training. A little later they reversed themselves and decided that under exceptional conditions credit might be given for foreign training. The candidate in question who precipitated this reversal had trained for two years with Sir (later Lord) Russell Brock.

Near the end of the decade the American Association for Thoracic Surgery made a decision that any candidate for membership must be certified by the Board of Thoracic Surgery. There were a few outstanding leaders in the field of cardiovascular surgery who did not have their *Boards* in thoracic surgery. It was decided that these surgeons could be excepted from the standard requirements and take just the oral examination. They included such stellar figures as Drs. Harris B Shumacker, Ormand Julian, Charles Hufnagel, and William Glenn. (As you might expect, they all passed, were certified, and became members of the AATS.)

Relations with the American Board of Surgery

Relations with the American Board of Surgery were amicable for the most part. A serious difference of opinion occurred only once. The

AT ONE THORACIC BOARD MEETING, AFTER A REPRESENTATIVE OF THE ABS HAD PRESENTED THEIR NEW RULES AND LEFT, THERE WAS HEATED DISCUSSION AND THE SUGGESTION WAS MADE THAT IT MIGHT BE DESIRABLE TO SEPARATE FROM THE AMERICAN BOARD OF SURGERY.

American Board of Surgery had changed certain training requirements which affected trainees desiring to enter training in thoracic surgery. At issue was the length of the training and the point at which a candidate could take the certifying examination. At one thoracic board meeting, after a representative of the ABS had presented their new rules and left, there was heated discussion and the suggestion was made that it might be desirable to separate from the American Board of Surgery. The Board of Thoracic Surgery felt they were being discriminated against. The changes suggested by the ABS were never implemented.

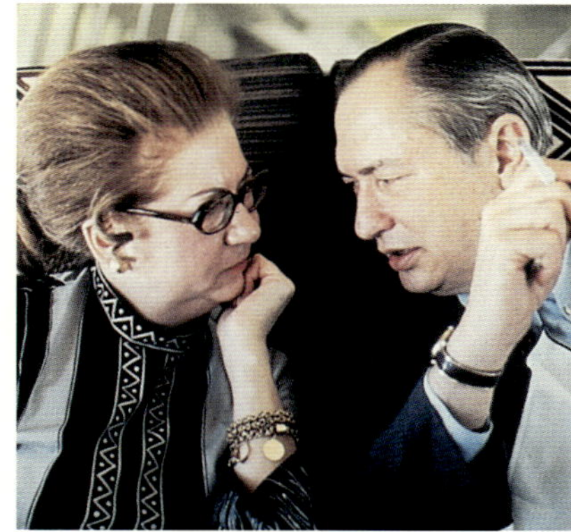

Louise Sper and Dr. Ralph Alley, Board member from 1969–1975, working in flight.

Beginning to Deal with Training Programs

Thereafter, a great deal more attention began to be paid to the problem of training program approval. At the May 1952 meeting, Dr. Tuttle reviewed the entire history of training program approval from the establishment of the Board to the present. He reported in detail the changes in attitude of the Board concerning the approval of hospitals for residency training in thoracic surgery, the manner in which the Committee on Resident Training had functioned since its inception, and the present status of the formation of a Conference Committee with the American College of Surgeons. There was further discussion of the amount of credit that should be given for preceptor training. After considerable discussion, the Board concluded that the individual case should be decided on its merits, with particular attention paid to the individual providing the training and his recommendations.

1961 Examination fee is raised to $125.

1963 Mixed training programs are no longer approved. Pressure from ABMS for BTS to separate from ABS mounts.

1966 The Board considers the establishment of a bipartite residency review committee.

During this time one of the less intellectual events in Board history occurred. It had been the practice of Dr. Joseph Gale, who hailed from Madison, to bring various Wisconsin cheeses to the Board meetings. He could not be present at one particular meeting but sent the cheeses with his associate, Dr. Anthony Curreri. Several of the Board members, who shall remain nameless, sent Dr. Gale a telegram saying "Evarts Graham desperately ill with botulism. Hope it isn't the cheese." Dr. Graham had been Dr. Gale's mentor.

Dr. Gale was so concerned that he routed out a medical librarian at an ungodly hour and checked out a book on toxicology. He learned that botulism could be carried by cheese. Dr. Graham later wrote, at the end of a letter, "P.S. I am about recovered from the botulism."

Focus on Cardiovascular Surgery

In their further consideration of training, the Board looked at a number of other issues: For example, they believed training programs should be broadened and should include experience in cardiovascular surgery. The Board previously had not examined a candidate on cardiovascular surgery if he had not been exposed to this area. Now, in 1956, the Board felt that a candidate should be examined in the field, whatever his experience. There was acceptance of the idea that the Board should establish jurisdiction over cardiovascular surgery by examining in the field. There was a general belief that it was desirable to have members of the Board who had cardiovascular experience.

THE BOARD BELIEVED TRAINING PROGRAMS SHOULD BE BROADENED AND SHOULD INCLUDE EXPERIENCE IN CARDIOVASCULAR SURGERY. THERE WAS A GENERAL BELIEF THAT IT WAS DESIRABLE TO HAVE MEMBERS OF THE BOARD WHO HAD CARDIOVASCULAR EXPERIENCE.

They also agreed that the director of a thoracic surgery training program should have achieved training in both thoracic and cardiovascular surgery and be certified by the Board of Thoracic Surgery. The Board was warned that this might result in legal action, but they held their ground and only implied there might be exceptional circumstances in which an outstanding individual might direct a program without being certified by the Board. In further discussion of "mixed" programs (programs where general surgery and thoracic surgery were mixed together into one program (often in some of the best academic medical centers) it was recognized that these were of several types. While some provided satisfactory training, others were clearly inadequate. Eventually mixed programs were no longer approved. Preceptor training also was no longer approved.

As a result of the decreasing tuberculosis patient load and the increasing volume of cardiovascular surgery, a questionnaire was sent to all directors of approved training programs in thoracic surgery inquiring whether cardiovascular surgery was included in the residency training program and, if so, what proportion of cases it represented.

Dr. William Adams analyzed the responses and determined that, in 35 institutions, relatively little cardiovascular work was being done by most of the residents. In a very few institutions a resident might have performed 30 or more cardiac or vascular procedures in a year. In a letter to Dr. John Jones, Dr. Burford commented that while most

IN THESE ONGOING DISCUSSIONS THE BOARD ALSO CONSIDERED THAT THEY HAD CHANGED THEIR ATTITUDE TOWARD PROGRAM APPROVAL. IN THE BEGINNING THE BOARD HAD BELIEVED THEY SHOULD NOT BE INVOLVED IN THIS ACTIVITY, BUT AS TIME WENT ON, THEY HAD COME TO ACCEPT THE RESPONSIBILITY.

training programs included cardiovascular surgery, the volume was nowhere near as much as might be expected from the barroom chatter of some people.

Establishment of the Residency Review Committee

Starting in 1953 and throughout the 1950s and 1960s, continuing attention was paid to the problem of program approval and the establishment of a tripartite residency review committee. The Council on Medical Education of the AMA, the American College of Surgeons, and the Board of Thoracic Surgery conducted discussions throughout those several years, and these were reported at Board meetings as *status quo*, the stumbling block apparently lying with the American College of Surgeons.

In these ongoing discussions the Board also considered that they had changed their attitude toward program approval. In the beginning the Board had believed they should not be involved in this activity, but as time went on, they had come to accept the responsibility. Having begun to deal with the problem of preceptor training as well as the mixed residencies, at almost every meeting these programs were discussed and many were disapproved. From the beginning the Board emphasized the need for two years of training to include both tuberculosis and non-tuberculosis patients.

1967 The Tripartite Residency Review Ccmmittee for Thoracic Surgery is approved on March 10, 1967.

1968 Experimental training programs, peripheral vascular surgery as part of general surgery, and cardiac surgery as part of thoracic surgery are discussed.

There was particular concern about programs in Veterans Hospitals. Personnel changed frequently and case distribution was often limited. The Board decided to require yearly statements about the program director and clinical activity from these hospitals.

In the middle of 1966, the Board considered the establishment of a bipartite residency review committee. Upon hearing this, the ACS reopened the issue of a tripartite committee. Dr. Paul Samson, a Regent of the College, and Drs. David Dugan and Donald Paulson, supported the ACS proposal, and after several more months of negotiations, the tripartite Residency Review Committee for Thoracic Surgery was finally approved on March 10, 1967.

Dr. Hiram T. Langston and Dr. Donald B. Effler accepted appointments by the Regents to be representatives of the College on the new committee. They met for the first time April 19, 1967, with the representatives of the AMA Council on Medical Education being Dr. Henry T. Bahnson and Dr. John W. Strieder. Dr. Edward J. Beattie, Jr., and Dr. James V. Maloney, Jr., represented the Board of Thoracic Surgery. Dr. John Nunemaker and Dr. Willard Thompson, of the AMA Council staff, and Dr. Stephenson representing the College, were also present.

1964–1969 Dr. Beattie chairs ad hoc committee to look at matching programs for residents through the American Board of Medical Specialties.

1969 ABMS recommends that BTS become a primary Board. Exam fee is raised to $250. Trial training programs to be established. Two more representatives from STS are accepted.

During early meetings of this committee there was clarification of requirements identifying experience in thoracic surgery, and a demand that all approved programs provide complete training, through established affiliations if necessary.

It was during this time also, that agitation for a matching program for residents began. Dr. Beattie chaired an ad hoc committee to look at matching programs for residents through the American Board of Medical Specialties from 1964–1969. It was a long process, however, and a matching program for thoracic surgery residents didn't come to fruition until 1992, under the aegis of the Thoracic Surgery Directors Association.

Essentials of Adequate Training Developed

The question of just what constituted adequate thoracic surgery training arose as a natural result of these changes. A Resident Training Committee was established by the Board of Thoracic Surgery, and Dr. Julian Johnson was assigned the responsibility of developing a statement about adequate training. These essentials were approved by the Board and later published in the Journal of the American Medical Association.

The preliminary draft of this document included the following concepts:

DURING EARLY MEETINGS OF THE RESIDENCY REVIEW COMMITTEE, THERE WAS CLARIFICATION OF REQUIREMENTS IDENTIFYING EXPERIENCE IN THORACIC SURGERY, AND A DEMAND THAT ALL APPROVED PROGRAMS PROVIDE COMPLETE TRAINING, THROUGH ESTABLISHED AFFILIATIONS IF NECESSARY.

Introduction

- Thoracic surgery residencies should be so organized as to provide tutelage in all aspects of thoracic diseases, intimately relating pathology and the basic sciences to clinical experience. Endoscopic experience is considered basic.

- The surgical experience must encompass two years of progressively graded responsibility, likewise, as nearly as possible, in all aspects of the field.

- To achieve this, affiliation between complementing services or institutions and utilization of cardiopulmonary laboratories as well as research facilities are to be encouraged.

- The purpose of such a program is to so train the resident that he (or she) will be adjudged by the Board of Thoracic Surgery, after examination, to be capable of safely pursuing professional growth by independent practice.

Prerequisites

- The candidate for training must be qualified for examination by the American Board of Surgery or be so qualified at the conclusion of a specified period of training in thoracic surgery. A candidate cannot be admitted to the examination of the Board of Thoracic Surgery without being certified by the American Board of Surgery.

"WHERE THE THORACIC SURGICAL EXPERIENCE IS OBTAINED ON A PROGRAM WHICH INTEGRATES GENERAL AND THORACIC SURGERY, THE ADEQUACY OF THIS EXPERIENCE MUST BE EVALUATED ON AN INDIVIDUAL BASIS."

Duration of Training

- A minimum of two years must be spent in this training during which time the candidate's surgical experience should by preference be exclusively in the field of thoracic disease and the 24 months should by preference be consecutive. Rotations should occur no oftener than every four months and preferably not oftener than every six months.

- Where the thoracic surgical experience is obtained on a program which integrates general and thoracic surgery, the adequacy of this experience must be evaluated on an individual basis.

Scope of Training

- The training must be so planned as to fulfill the following objectives:
  a. Thorough understanding of the basic sciences as they apply to thoracic surgery.
  b. Graded and progressive assumption of operative responsibility.
  c. Finally, assumption of total responsibility for the patient's care in all its aspects under proper supervision.

This preliminary draft, which shows how seriously the Board took its responsibilities along with their vision of thoracic surgical training, then went on to encourage affiliations between diverse services in order to assure experience in all aspects of the field, since few hospitals were capable of providing this experience. It noted that experience gained on purely private services could not form the basis of a

IT WAS NOTED THAT EXPERIENCE GAINED ON PURELY PRIVATE SERVICES COULD NOT FORM THE BASIS OF A TRAINING PROGRAM. FINALLY, PRECEPTORSHIPS AND PRECEPTOR-TYPE TRAINING WERE DEEMED NOT ACCEPTABLE.

training program. Finally, preceptorships and preceptor-type training were deemed not acceptable.

The draft underwent revision and was finally accepted by the Board. It represented an ideal which, in many ways, became the accepted form of thoracic training.

Name Change Considered

The Journal of Thoracic Surgery had changed its title to *The Journal of Thoracic and Cardiovascular Surgery* in 1959. The programs of the AATS were being dominated by cardiovascular papers. The question arose as to whether the Board should also change its name. There were pros and cons among the many interested parties, including the AATS, the American College of Surgeons, the American Heart Association, the ABS, the AMA, and others. At this time there was a struggle in the Surgical Section of the AMA over control of this body. While there was acceptance of a name change for the Board by many, it was finally decided that this probably was not an appropriate time to try to accomplish this goal.

The struggle within the Surgical Section of the AMA also had an unintended consequence. Dr. Robert Shaw and his wife had accepted an opportunity to work in Afghanistan with MEDICO. This meant that Dr. Shaw would be leaving before his term as a Board member was completed. Because he had been appointed to the Board by the AMA, it was decided that no replacement for him would be requested until the battle within the Surgical Section of the AMA was over.

AMONG THE SUGGESTIONS TO A QUERY ABOUT THIS WAS, FOR THE FIRST TIME, ONE THAT THE BOARD MIGHT BECOME INDEPENDENT FROM THE AMERICAN BOARD OF SURGERY. AT THIS POINT, SOME OF THE BOARD MEMBERS WERE NOT READY TO ACCEPT SUCH A SUGGESTION.

Although he looked forward to his service in Afghanistan, Dr. Shaw evidently must have had some regrets about leaving the Board. In a letter to Dr. Tuttle, written as he was leaving, he said, "I agree with John Strieder when he says that it (the Board) is the 'best club' to which he has ever belonged."

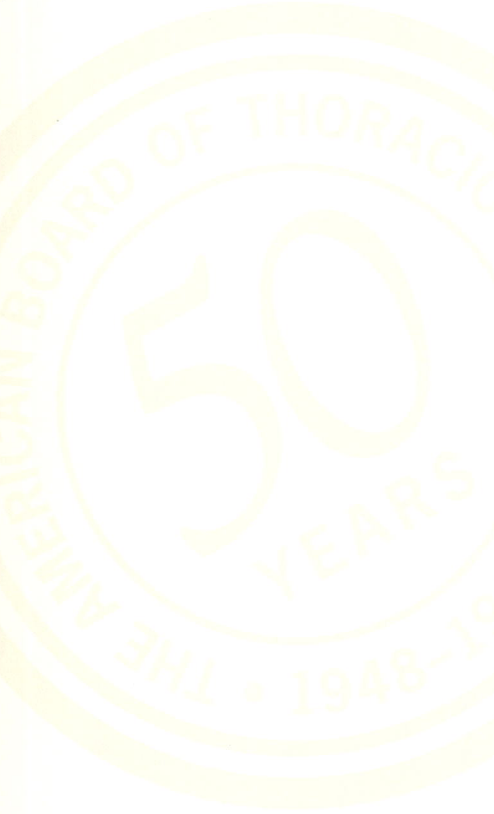

Impact of Medical Politics

The political world of specialties was also becoming more complicated. The Advisory Board for Medical Specialties, which became the American Board of Medical Specialties in 1971, was coming into being. Because the Board was an affiliate of the American Board of Surgery, it did not have representation on this body. Among the suggestions to a query about this was, for the first time, one that the Board might become independent from the American Board of Surgery. At this point, some of the Board members were not ready to accept such a suggestion.

Budget Increases

Increasing Board expenses finally required raising the examination fee to $125 in 1961. An auditing firm had been employed. Meetings were recorded by a stenographer. By this time a member of the Board was also accepted as a member of the ABS, although he did not participate in the examinations.

Board members did submit questions for the written part of the ABS examination. In the written Part I examination of the ABS,

DR. TUTTLE WAS A TREMENDOUSLY IMPORTANT FIGURE IN THE DEVELOPMENT OF THE BOARD. NO ONE COULD HAVE BEEN MORE DEDICATED TO ITS FUTURE. WITH HIS DEATH [IN **1962**] AN ERA CAME TO AN END.

40–45% of the questions related to thoracic surgery. During this time period arrangements had been made for thoracic surgery candidates to take Part I of the general surgery boards in lieu of a written thoracic surgery examination. The ABS turned to a multiple choice examination and this stimulated the Board to reevaluate its own examination.

Changing of the Guard

In December 1962, Dr. Tuttle died after an extended illness. Dr. Clagett was elected Secretary in a conference call. This brought to an end an important influence on the Board. Despite his sometimes rough demeanor and forceful and intimidating personality, he was a tremendously important figure in the development of the Board. No one could have been more dedicated to its future. With his death an era came to an end.

CHAPTER 5

The Modern Era

1966 Millis Commission Report on the surgical specialties is completed.

1967 The first meeting of the tripartite Residency Review Committee (RRC) is conducted.

The years between 1963 and 1973 marked another distinct period in the Board's history. Cardiac surgery was coming into its own, and the specialty of thoracic surgery had carved a distinct place for itself in the annals of medical history.

FERMENT AND CHANGE IN THE EXAMINATION

Two men served as Board Secretary during this very significant period: O. Theron Clagett and Rollin Daniel, both of whom had previously served very effectively as Chairman. The Board Chairmen during this time were: John Strieder, Rollin Daniel, Edward Beattie, David Dugan, and Donald Paulson, all of whom provided strong leadership. This was a time of ferment in the world of specialties and certification. The Millis Report (*see* **Appendix A**), among others, was critical of graduate medical education.

The Thoracic Board Examination

Major changes in the thoracic Board examination and in training requirements were made as well. In the early days of the Board, examiners brought their own x-rays to the examination. They were not above using "trick" x-rays to confound the candidate. As an example,

1970 Oral examination is restructured with professional assistance. Office moves to East Detroit.

1971 On January 1, ABTS becomes an independent primary member board of the ABMS.

Julian Johnson brought the x-ray of a tightly corseted woman whose waist was the size of her neck and displayed it to the candidates upside down. The only candidate he examined who interpreted the film correctly that day was Timothy Takaro.

In the sixties there was a move to standardize this part of the examination by duplicating the x-rays used so that each examiner employed the same set of films. Ted Beattie spearheaded this effort, which greatly improved the quality of the oral examination. Handling these films finally became the responsibility of Dave Dugan, but he was faced with transporting a huge file of films to the examination site. This problem he solved by having a special box built to hold them. To aid in their transportation he attached one of his children's skateboards to the box. This brought him all kinds of attention from airline stewardesses (as they were known in those days). Who knows but that Dr. Dugan's "baggage on a skateboard" may have inspired the current epidemic of "pull behind" luggage seen at every airport today.

Dr. Fred Kittle, who served on the Board from 1967–1975 recalls how difficult x-rays and challenging pathological specimens shown in the morning by Jim Clagett, his immediate predecessor as Examination Chairman, became universally recognized by the end of the day. Such cross-contamination was abrogated by abolishing the projected pathology slides and substantially changing the oral examination method.

1972 Self-assessment exam is discussed. Oral examination changes to four separate examiners.

1973 Minimum case guidelines are approved, bylaws are modified. Failed candidates can have hearing.

The first revised oral examination was a complicated schedule on a large brown piece of paper that shocked Louise Sper when she saw it. Fundamentally, it was designed so that each candidate was asked the same questions during the morning with a different set of equal significance for those examined in the afternoon. Questions and their desired answers were supplied to the examiners to obviate individual preferences/biases by the examiners. A traffic pattern was devised so that communication between those examined and those to be examined was eliminated.

In the midst of all these exam changes, Dr. Kittle added a famous photograph to the archives of Board history: Modeled after a satirical 1811 drawing by G. Cruickshank that ridicules the examination process at the Royal College of Surgeons, Dr. Kittle's photograph substitutes thoracic surgery lights of the 1970s (*see pages 72–73*).

The Board began to consider administering its own written examination, following the lead of the American Board of Surgery, which was employing a multiple choice question examination. The Thoracic Board developed their own multiple choice question exam, and a professional firm was employed to assist in this effort. Board members all helped provide questions for the examination. Careful preparations to administer the first of these examinations were made to avoid any mistakes. When the examination booklets were collected, the examination administrator realized that one was missing and, after checking, it was concluded that an extra booklet had been handed out. At

Describe, the Organs of Hearing.
you paid too dear for it brother Sergent.
The EXAMINATION, of a YOUNG SURGEON.

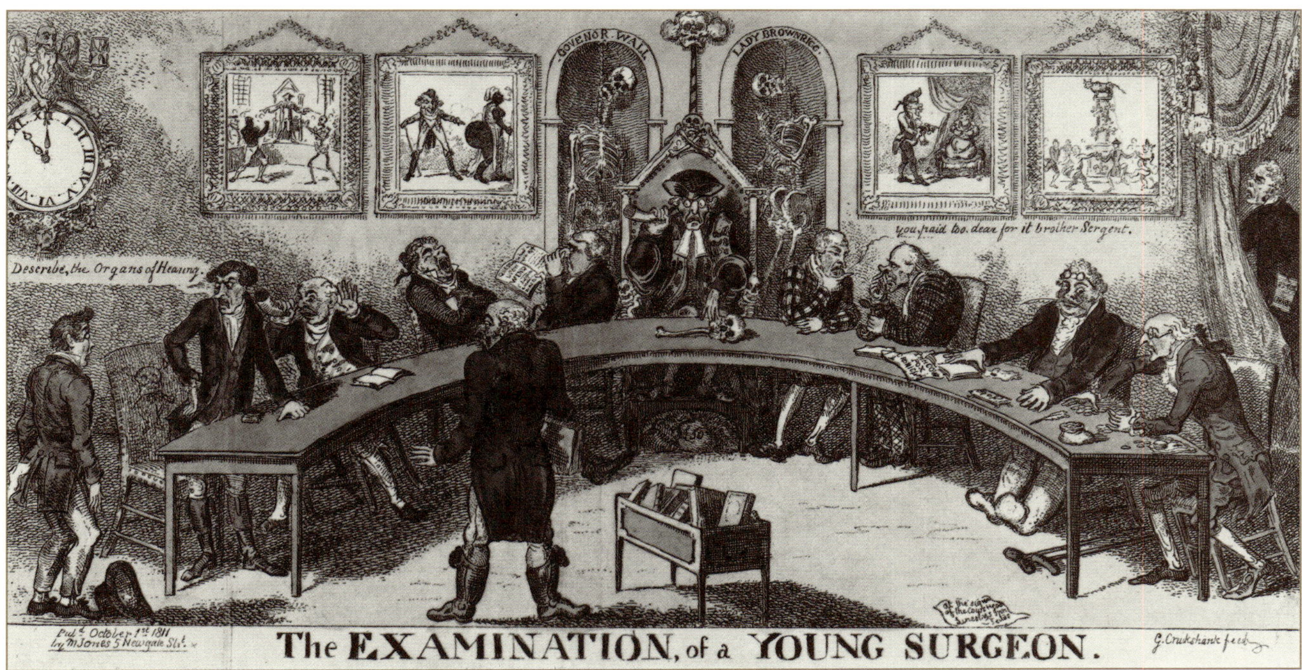

G. Cruickshank's satirical drawing of an examination being conducted at the Royal College of Surgeons in 1811.

that point there was nothing to be done. The booklet was returned by mail to the Board office a few days later. It had been opened.

One interesting sidelight to the written examination was the change in smoking habits. Most of the written examinations were administered in one large room, usually in Dallas, with many rows of tables at which the examinees sat. The examination was obviously a time of great stress, and at first many of the candidates smoked. As the years went by, the number of smokers steadily decreased until only a table or two was reserved for the few remaining smokers.

FROM AFFILIATE TO INDEPENDENT

The most important change in the status of the Board occurred when they moved from being an affiliate of the American Board of Surgery to being a primary board. This change was first suggested in 1969 when it was noted that the Board of Thoracic Surgery was the only affiliate Board. The Advisory Board of Medical Specialties (which became the American Board of Medical Specialties in 1971) had also suggested that the Board should become primary if they wished to have a vote in their medical specialties forum.

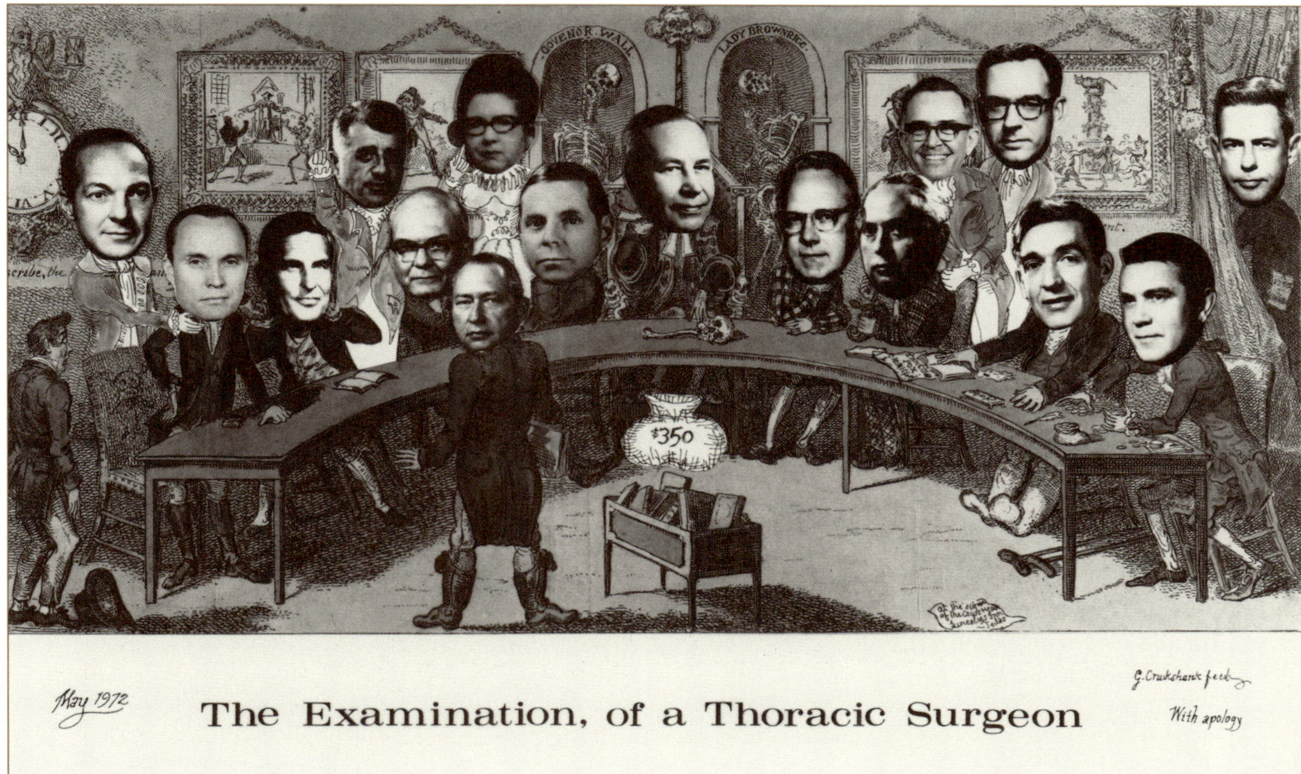

An American Board of Thoracic Surgery examination, à la Cruickshank.

Left to right:
Dr. Jay Ankeney, Dr. James Malm, Dr. Ben Roe, Dr. Hans Ehrenhaft, Dr. Will Sealy, Dr. Ralph Alley, Louise Sper, Dr. F. Henry Ellis, Dr. Donald Paulson, Dr. Herbert Sloan, Dr. Myron Wheat, Dr. Robert Ellison, Dr. Tom Ferguson, Dr. Fred Kittle, Dr. Paul Adkins, Dr. Rollin Daniel.

The ABMS approved ABTS as a member Board in 1970, and the ABTS became an independent primary member board of the ABMS on January 1, 1971, at which time the word American was added to its name. A revised certificate was offered to all Diplomates of the Board of Thoracic Surgery at a cost of $50, and many accepted the offer. The revised certificate incorporated these changes:

1. A change in the name of the organization.
2. Elimination of "An Affiliate of the American Board of Surgery."
3. A change in the certifying statement on the certificate to:

"The American Board of Thoracic Surgery created in 1948 for the certification of Thoracic Surgeons hereby declares that ___________ name ___________ having satisfied all the requirements and successfully passed the examination is hereby awarded the Board's certificate in the specialty of Thoracic and Cardiac Surgery."

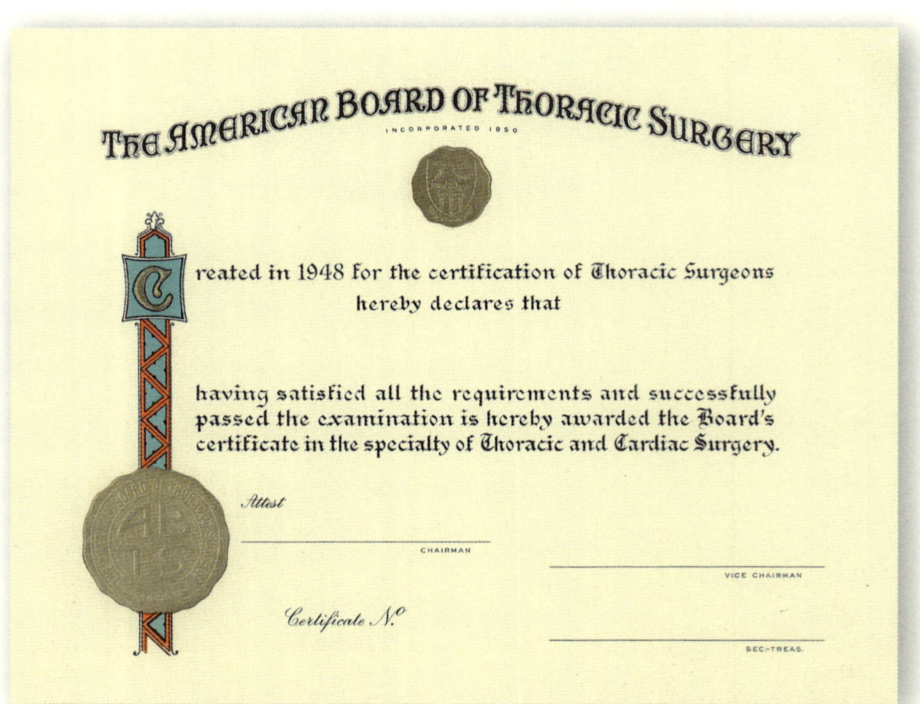

THE AMERICAN BOARD OF THORACIC SURGERY

INCORPORATED 1950

Created in 1948 for the certification of Thoracic Surgeons
hereby declares that

having satisfied all the requirements and successfully passed the examination is hereby awarded the Board's certificate in the specialty of Thoracic and Cardiac Surgery.

Attest

CHAIRMAN

VICE CHAIRMAN

Certificate No

SEC.-TREAS.

Revised certificate for the American Board of Thoracic Surgery.

Changes in the certificate also brought it into line with criteria established by the American Board of Medical Specialties.

More Changes

As the decade came to a close, several events occurred, some more important than others. In an effort to control the sometimes rambunctious members of the Board, the Chairman, Donald Paulson, employed a "clicker" to gain attention. At his retirement he was given a gold clicker to memorialize this addition to Roberts Rules of Order.

Another "first" instituted by Dr. Paulson was at the pre-meeting dinner. When it became necessary to do two or three hours worth of work in advance of the Board meeting the next day, Dr. Paulson cut off serving alcohol at dinner time. The distressed Board members, who were certain that they were as sharp as ever after an "enjoyable" dinner, were amazed to see their productivity improve substantially during the evening session.

THE BOARD HAD CLEARLY ESTABLISHED ITS INTEREST IN CARDIOVASCULAR SURGERY, AND THIS HAD BEEN ACCEPTED BY THE OTHER BODIES INTERESTED IN CARDIAC AND VASCULAR PROBLEMS.

To Be or Not to Be a Cardiovascular Board

The Board had clearly established its interest in cardiovascular surgery, and this had been accepted by the other bodies interested in cardiac and vascular problems. Discussions of a separate cardiovascular board had never led to any serious move to accomplish this. Within the Board there was far-reaching conversation about the inclusion of the term *cardiovascular* in its name. At times the discussions were somewhat heated. Finally, the text of the certificate was revised to state that the holder was qualified in cardiac surgery.

Mark Ravitch, a Hopkins legend who taught me much of what I knew, wrote a critical letter to the Board wondering how he could suddenly be certified in cardiac surgery when he did none. This small brouhaha quickly blew over.

THE BOARD OFFICE MOVES AND GROWS

Changes were also occurring in the administration of the Board. For many years the Board had enjoyed rent-free space in the Herman Kiefer Hospital. Problems in Detroit, including the riots in 1967, which occurred close to the hospital, made it desirable to move the office. In 1970, suitable space was found in a professional building in East Detroit. At the same time, the amount of work in the office was increasing and additional help became necessary. The increase in the number of candidates also increased expenses. Everyone realized that higher examination fees could not meet all needs, and the Board

1974 Self-assessment examination is given. 100 case experience is accepted for candidates.

1976 Candidates must complete approved program.

decided to request $7,500 a year from each of the two thoracic surgical societies. In 1976 this amount was raised to $10,000 per year. Considerable discussion ensued about the need to remain independent of the societies, but it was finally decided to make the requests, which were granted. Support from the societies continued for many years in increasing amounts, ultimately amounting to $25,000 from each. Finally, in 1985, diplomate fees were raised to $1,000 which would cover the expenses of the Board office, and support from the two societies was terminated.

Special Meetings Called

Two special meetings of the Board were held during this time. The first was held on February 6, 1966, and the second on May 25, 1969. They were convened to address special problems outside normal Board agendas. During the 1966 meeting, the group voted to eliminate straight, one-year residencies. As previously mentioned, the Board had also agreed to accept the invitation to help the AMA Council on Medical Education to participate in a tripartite Residency Review Committee (RRC) for Thoracic Surgery. Agreement was finally reached, and the first meeting of this tripartite committee occurred in 1967. Thereafter, the RRC was responsible for evaluating programs. The last action of this meeting was to approve the addition of two Board members from the Society of Thoracic Surgeons.

MIXED PROGRAMS WERE NO LONGER APPROVED DESPITE THE FEELING BY MEMBERS FROM UNIVERSITY CENTERS (WHERE MOST OF THE PROGRAMS WERE LOCATED) THAT THE QUALITY OF MEN (THERE WERE NO WOMEN RESIDENTS YET) WAS OFTEN SUPERIOR TO CANDIDATES FROM APPROVED PROGRAMS.

Three years later in 1969, at a fall Board meeting, the number of representatives from the Society of Thoracic Surgeons was increased to four. The Board decided that a reevaluation of examining procedures was necessary. Heretofore, certification in thoracic surgery had required previous certification in general surgery followed by two years experience in thoracic surgery. An alternative proposal was made whereby three years of general surgery that did not lead to certification would be followed by three years of thoracic surgery. It was suggested that this program would lead to a better trained thoracic surgeon.

OTHER CHANGES IN TRAINING

Other changes in the training process took place during these years. Mixed programs were no longer approved despite the feeling by members from university centers (where most of the programs were located) that the quality of men (there were no women residents yet) was often superior to candidates from approved programs. Most Board members accepted this but recognized that evaluating these programs was difficult. Thus they concluded that program directors in these institutions should apply for an approved program. This recommendation was forwarded on to the RRC.

A total of five centers had been approved for the new three-and-three trial program. The hope was that as many as 10 to 15 of these programs might be established. A few trainees completed the program, but it finally died from lack of interest. Although the new

IT WAS NECESSARY TO TEACH THE RESIDENTS TECHNICAL SKILLS THAT SHOULD HAVE BEEN ACQUIRED IN GENERAL SURGERY.

program demonstrated that a well-trained thoracic surgeon could be produced in this way, several elements made the standard program more desirable:

1. In spite of promises, the three-and-three trainees did not receive the training in general surgery which they had been told they would get, at least in one of the programs.
2. It was necessary to teach the residents technical skills that should have been acquired in general surgery.
3. Many residents were interested in vascular surgery and thus wanted to be certified in general surgery as an initial step.
4. In one center rivalry grew up between the special residents and those progressing through the standard program.

As an alternative to defining the "ideal surgical training program," Donald Effler suggested that it consist of:

1. A six year program satisfying both the requirements of general surgery and thoracic surgery.
2. Limitation of laboratory work to six months.
3. Training in every part of thoracic and cardiovascular surgery.
4. Training exclusively under the direction of one program director.

Board members were in general agreement with these principles. Gordon Scannell also agreed but noted that, while one year of thoracic surgery might be credited to general surgery, the senior year of thoracic surgery should be exclusively thoracic.

THE MILLIS REPORT RECOMMENDED THAT A COMMISSION ON GRADUATE EDUCATION BE ESTABLISHED TO PLAN, COORDINATE, AND REVIEW STANDARDS FOR GRADUATE MEDICAL EDUCATION.

IMPACT OF THE MILLIS REPORT ON MEDICAL EDUCATION

Dr. Edward Beattie reported to the Board on October 6, 1967, on a meeting of the Surgical Specialty Boards hosted by the American Board of Orthopedic Surgery. One aim had been to consider the impact of the Millis Commission Report (*see* **Appendix A**) on the surgical specialties.

Dr. Beattie summarized the changes that had occurred in graduate medical education since the Millis Report in 1966:

1. The internship was abolished.
2. The Advisory Board of Medical Specialties was abolished and replaced by the American Board of Medical Specialties, which was dedicated to the development of more uniform requirements for specialty certification and greater cooperation among the many bodies involved in graduate medical education, particularly the specialty boards. The Advisory Board had been previously criticized as a federation of independent specialty boards with little control over the policies of its member boards or residency review committees.
3. The new emphasis on primary care had resulted in the establishment of the American Board of Family Practice.
4. The Report recommended that a Commission on Graduate Education be established to plan, coordinate, and review standards for graduate medical education. The major medical organizations had had extensive discussions about the proposal, but it had not yet been implemented.

IN THE MONTHS FOLLOWING THE RELEASE OF MILLIS, THE BOARD APPROVED THE DEVELOPMENT AND ADMINISTRATION OF AN IN-TRAINING EXAMINATION. THERE WAS VIGOROUS SUPPORT FOR VOLUNTARY RECERTIFICATION AND FOR A SELF-ASSESSMENT EXAMINATION.

He also reported on a statement formulated by the Graduate Education Committee of the American College of Surgeons to be submitted to the Board of Regents. This presumably would represent the position of the ACS, and it supported a number of positions including:

1. Elimination of the internship as a separate entity but including it as a part of the whole of graduate medical education.
2. Permitting flexibility, experimentation, and innovation in graduate medical education.
3. Reconstituting the Advisory Board of Medical Specialties to include other organizations concerned directly with graduate education, and granting it more responsibility and authority.

Board Changes Following Millis

In spite of its visionary goals, in many ways the Millis Report had less direct impact on the Thoracic Board than it did on other specialties, except perhaps in their relations with the hierarchy of graduate medical education.

Nevertheless, it influenced either directly or indirectly a number of important changes. In the months following the release of Millis, the Board approved the development and administration of an in-training examination. There was vigorous support for voluntary recertification and for a self-assessment examination.

THE BOARD BECAME CONCERNED THAT SOME CANDIDATES HAD INADEQUATE OPERATIVE EXPERIENCE....OVER TIME THIS STIMULATED PROGRAM DIRECTORS TO PROVIDE AN INCREASING VOLUME OF OPERATIVE EXPERIENCE TO THEIR RESIDENTS.

As the Board examined the operative experience that candidates obtained during their training, they became concerned that some candidates had what the Board held was inadequate experience. Long discussions occurred about what constituted adequate operative experience, but no specific number could be agreed to. James Maloney finally proposed that candidates with operative experience below the 30th percentile of the experience of all candidates should have their applications examined individually by the Credentials Committee. Over time this stimulated program directors to provide an increasing volume of operative experience to their residents.

LEADERSHIP CHANGES

"Jim" Clagett resigned as Board Secretary in 1967. One of the country's outstanding thoracic surgeons, he had a warm personality and was admired by all with whom he came in contact. He had been the obvious person to follow Bill Tuttle, and had been very important in lending strength to the Board when it embarked on the national graduate medical education scene. He was replaced by Rollin Daniel who had just completed his term as Chairman. Rollin brought extensive experience in medical administration as well as fine surgical credentials.

Rollin Daniel served extremely well during a time of expanding Board activity. He submitted his resignation in the Fall of 1972. I resigned as Vice-Chairman and was appointed Secretary-Treasurer in 1973, a position which I held through 1986.

CHAPTER 6

Challenges of the Seventies and Eighties

1974 Self-assessment examination is given. 100 case experience is accepted for candidates.

1975 IRS tax exempt classification changes from 501(c)3 to 501(c)6.

Louise Sper retired in 1986, which was also my last year as Secretary. I had worked alongside six Chairmen: Frederick Kittle, Paul Adkins, Thomas Ferguson, Robert Ellison, Benson Roe, Donald Mulder, and Hassan Najafi. All served during a time when they faced major problems and changes.

THE BOARD FACES MAJOR PROBLEMS

What were these problems? They ranged from finances through examining and certifying for general vascular surgery experience to recertification to relocation of the Board when Mrs. Sper retired. Among the major issues was the growing difficulty of dealing with the burgeoning bureaucracy and increasingly complicated alphabet soup of committees related to graduate medical education, that is: the Liaison Committee for Medical Education (LCME); the Liaison Committee for Graduate Medical Education (LCGME); the Coordinating Council for Continuing Medical Education (CCCME), the Accreditation Council for Graduate Medical Education (ACGME), and more. The Board meetings lengthened and the amount of paper devoted to the minutes increased as there were more and more committees reporting. Some of these were standing committees, some related to the outside world

THE BASIC CONCEPTS OF TRAINING AND CERTIFYING THORACIC SURGEONS WERE TO ESTABLISH A BASIC LEVEL OF COMPETENCE WHICH ALL TRAINEES MUST REACH, TO UNDERSTAND THAT DETERMINATION OF COMPETENCY REQUIRES MULTIPLE AREAS OF EVALUATION, AND TO PROVIDE CONTINUING EVALUATION.

of graduate medical education, and some were ad hoc committees appointed to deal with particular problems.

It was necessary to submit written committee reports before meetings, which occurred in the spring and fall, to include in the agendas. There were complaints about the rigidity of the format and the lack of meaningful discussion. Unfortunately, this seemed to be the only way to get through the ever-lengthening meetings.

In an effort to state the principles they had developed to train, examine, and certify thoracic surgeons, the Board published a position paper in the *Journal of Thoracic and Cardiovascular Surgery* in 1980.[1] The basic concepts were: (1) to establish a basic level of competence which all trainees must reach; (2) to understand that determination of competency requires multiple areas of evaluation; and (3) to provide continuing evaluation.

Competency was defined and measured and quality control ensured through at least four mechanisms. These included approved residency programs in thoracic surgery, certification by the American Board of Thoracic Surgery, state regulations, and local hospital regulations.

[1] *Journal of Thoracic and Cardiovascular Surgery*, 1980; 79:937.

CLINICAL COMPETENCE IN THORACIC SURGERY REQUIRES BOTH FACTUAL KNOWLEDGE AS WELL AS TECHNICAL SKILLS IN THE DIAGNOSIS AND TREATMENT OF PATHOLOGIC CONDITIONS INVOLVING THORACIC STRUCTURES.

In a letter dated November 9, 1978, to ABTS nominating organizations, a definition of competence in thoracic surgery was spelled out:

> *Clinical competence* in Thoracic Surgery requires both factual knowledge as well as technical skills in the diagnosis and treatment of pathologic conditions involving thoracic structures. Precise definition of the scope of thoracic surgery, as well as the current methods used to assess clinical competence, have been developed to be certain that an individual who is certified by the American Board of Thoracic Surgery has met certain standards of competency.
>
> The scope of thoracic surgery encompasses a knowledge of the normal and pathologic conditions of both cardiovascular and general thoracic structures. This involves all congenital and acquired lesions (including infections, trauma, tumors, and metabolic disorders) of both the heart and blood vessels, as well as those involving the lungs, pleura, chest wall, mediastinum, esophagus, and diaphragm. In addition, the ability to establish a precise diagnosis—an essential step toward proper therapy—requires familiarity with diagnostic procedures such as cardiac catheterization, angiography, electrocardiography, radiologic studies such as conventional and computerized tomography and imaging techniques, endoscopy, tissue biopsy and biologic and biochemical tests appropriate to thoracic diseases.

ANOTHER OF THE MANY IMPORTANT PROBLEMS THE BOARD WRESTLED WITH IN THE 1970S AND 1980S WAS THE QUESTION OF FINANCING THE INCREASINGLY EXPENSIVE CERTIFICATION PROCESS.

Finances

Another of the many important problems the Board wrestled with in the 1970s and 1980s was the question of financing the increasingly expensive certification process.

The Board recognized that its most important responsibility was certification of thoracic surgeons. However, this was becoming more and more costly as the examination procedures improved, and as the Board and its members spent more time relating to the outside world of graduate medical education.

Office expenses increased as the Board attempted to gain information about the candidates for certification and to analyze the performance of those candidates when they took the certifying examination. Sources of income, however, were limited. The first of these was the examination fee, but when this reached $1,000 for the certifying process, it was felt that the fee could not be raised beyond that level. Some income was also generated from selling examinations for such purposes as the In-Training Examination.

The two thoracic surgical societies continued to be extremely generous and made annual contributions to the Board, but the Board wished to be independent and not beholden to outside organizations. With Benson B. Roe, Charles Hatcher, and Harold Urschel taking the lead, discussions began on establishing an endowment fund. It was determined that such a fund would be tax exempt and that

AFTER DELIBERATIONS CONCERNING GENERAL VASCULAR SURGERY... THE BOARD HAD CLEARLY DECIDED NOT TO EXAMINE IN THE AREA OF GENERAL, NONTHORACIC VASCULAR, OR PERIPHERAL VASCULAR SURGERY.

contributions by diplomates would be deductible as a business expense. Starting in 1983, diplomates were solicited for an initial amount of $300 to be followed by a yearly contribution of $50. The response was good, and the fund rose above $1,000,000 in a relatively few years.

The Board had been concerned about financing Mrs. Sper's retirement, which was to occur in 1986. They did not want to repeat a problem that had occurred in another thoracic organization when a valued employee retired without a retirement program. Over the years the Board was able to establish a defined benefit plan for their two full-time employees. At the time of Louise Sper's retirement there were adequate funds in the plan, and the Board's financial status was solid.

Vascular Surgery

After deliberations concerning general vascular surgery by both the American Board of Surgery and the American Board of Thoracic Surgery, the Board had clearly decided not to examine in the area of general, nonthoracic vascular, or peripheral vascular surgery. However, several thoracic programs did provide excellent experience in general vascular surgery.

The question remained about how vascular surgery skills would be recognized. Discussions centered around a certificate of special competence in vascular surgery. Originally, there was opposition to such a

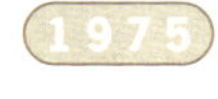
1975 D.O.'s accepted for examination if certified by ABS and have two years of training in approved program.

1976 Candidates must complete approved program.

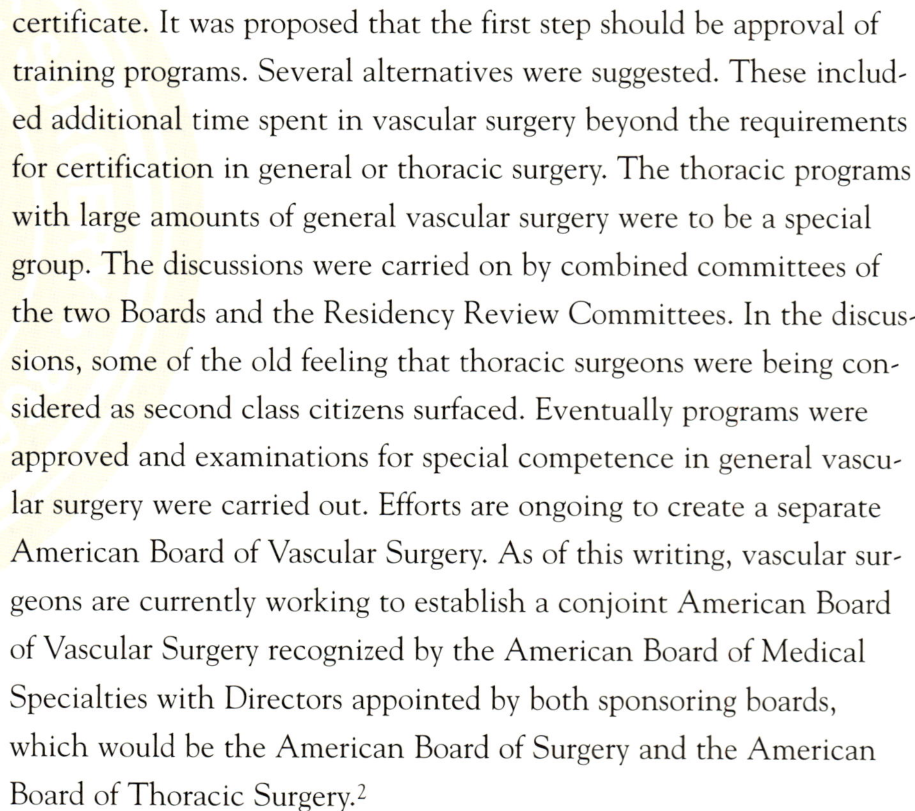

certificate. It was proposed that the first step should be approval of training programs. Several alternatives were suggested. These included additional time spent in vascular surgery beyond the requirements for certification in general or thoracic surgery. The thoracic programs with large amounts of general vascular surgery were to be a special group. The discussions were carried on by combined committees of the two Boards and the Residency Review Committees. In the discussions, some of the old feeling that thoracic surgeons were being considered as second class citizens surfaced. Eventually programs were approved and examinations for special competence in general vascular surgery were carried out. Efforts are ongoing to create a separate American Board of Vascular Surgery. As of this writing, vascular surgeons are currently working to establish a conjoint American Board of Vascular Surgery recognized by the American Board of Medical Specialties with Directors appointed by both sponsoring boards, which would be the American Board of Surgery and the American Board of Thoracic Surgery.[2]

At the AATS meeting in 1980, an informal group met to discuss the problem of training in general thoracic surgery. Figures were quoted showing that, in 1978, residents performed twice as many cardiac operations as general thoracic procedures. Experience in esophageal surgery, especially, was noted to be lacking.

---

[2] Stanley J., et al. The American Board of Vascular Surgery. *J Vasc Surg*, (in press, 1998).

DISCUSSION AT BOARD MEETINGS ABOUT RECERTIFICATION SURFACED IN THE EARLY 1970s. IT WAS ALREADY SPREADING AMONG THE OTHER MEMBER BOARDS IN THE AMERICAN BOARD OF MEDICAL SPECIALTIES.

In 1985 and 1986 there was discussion about critical care and who should deliver it. The American Board of Surgery wanted to obtain permission from The American Board of Medical Specialties to award a certificate of added qualifications in surgical critical care. The ABTS opposed this concept, believing that training in thoracic surgery included training in the postoperative care of thoracic surgical patients.

Competence in other related areas, such as endoscopy, emergency room management, and oncology also went unrecognized. This lack of recognition loomed later on as a problem and an erosion into the surgical "territory" by the medical proceduralists.

Recertification

Discussion at Board meetings about recertification surfaced in the early 1970s. It was already spreading among the other member boards in the American Board of Medical Specialties. This meant, of course, that certificates would be time-limited. In general, there was approval of the concept. Recertification was to include continuing medical education, practice audits, and either a cognitive examination or some sort of self-assessment. Voluntary recertification was already being offered by several boards.

In the early discussions there was a feeling that this was too large an undertaking for the Board, and that it should be handled by another body. The Board finally accepted the responsibility and reaffirmed the

IT WOULD BE NECESSARY FOR THE DIPLOMATES TO KEEP RECORDS OF CONTINUING MEDICAL EDUCATION AND OF OPERATIONS PERFORMED WITH MORTALITY RATES AND TO SUBMIT THESE RECORDS.

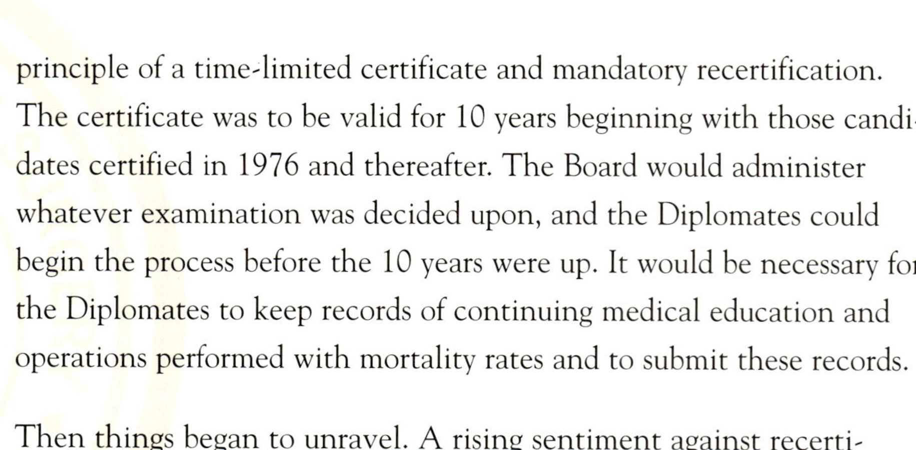

principle of a time-limited certificate and mandatory recertification. The certificate was to be valid for 10 years beginning with those candidates certified in 1976 and thereafter. The Board would administer whatever examination was decided upon, and the Diplomates could begin the process before the 10 years were up. It would be necessary for the Diplomates to keep records of continuing medical education and operations performed with mortality rates and to submit these records.

Then things began to unravel. A rising sentiment against recertification fomented in several boards. At meetings of the Society of Thoracic Surgeons, some members raised violent objections to this proposed intrusion into their independence and what they believed to be their inalienable rights. As importantly, opposition to recertification grew within the Board. On October 29, 1982, a motion was made to rescind the decision to offer a time-limited certificate. The vote was tied and the Chairman, Benson Roe, cast the deciding vote against the motion. Thereafter, recertification was not challenged and the process went forward.

Through the Coordinating Committee for Continuing Education in Thoracic Surgery (CCCETS—an acronym that aptly illustrates the alphabet soup committee structure), a syllabus was developed. Jay Ankeney was one of the moving forces in the effort to produce materials for self-learning and self-assessment.

1976 Practice of issuing time-limited certificates, valid for a period of 10 years, is implemented.

1977 First operations manual is prepared. Committee is established to consider requirements for graduate education in vascular surgery.

Requirements for recertification currently include:

1. Holding a certificate issued by the ABTS at the time of application for recertification. Expiration of this certificate would not disqualify a candidate for recertification.
2. Holding a currently valid license to practice medicine.
3. Submitting evidence of accumulation of 100 hours of approved postgraduate medical education during the two years preceding application.
4. Submitting a practice review in the form of an operative experience covering the most recent 100 consecutive major operations performed or, if the operative experience is less than 100 major cases in the most recent year, the total experience for the year should be submitted.

The diplomate was then to take a cognitive examination which he/she would be required to pass. On further consideration, mortality incidence figures were to be submitted but would have no impact on admission to the recertifying process. Nor was there to be a pass/fail examination. Instead, a Self-Evaluation/Self-Assessment Examination for Thoracic Surgery (SESATS) would be taken by the diplomate. Operative experience was reduced to one year.

THE THORACIC SURGERY DIRECTORS ASSOCIATION (TSDA) BECAME AN IMPORTANT LIAISON BETWEEN THE BOARD AND THE PROGRAM DIRECTORS. IT DEVELOPED FROM A SMALL BREAKFAST GRIPE SESSION TO AN EFFECTIVE AND DEDICATED ORGANIZATION.

THE THORACIC SURGERY DIRECTORS ASSOCIATION

In 1976 the Thoracic Surgery Directors Association (TSDA) first reported its activities to the Board. This organization became an important liaison between the Board and the program directors. It developed from a small breakfast gripe session to an effective and dedicated organization. A representative of the TSDA attended Board meetings on a regular basis, and the Vice-President of the Board attended TSDA meetings. This interface between the Board and the program directors grew increasingly important as time went on.

The program directors limited membership to directors of approved programs. They addressed the problems of inadequate programs, both in leadership and clinical case material. Concern was expressed about erosion of clinical material to other disciplines. The problem of what should be done with the inadequate resident was examined. Additionally, the problem of examining for congenital heart disease experience was discussed. An in-training examination was proposed and administered. This responsibility eventually was transferred to the Board, and they gave their first in-training exam in 1983. Finally, the TSDA undertook the beginnings of a matching plan for thoracic residents, which was finally implemented in 1992.

IN-TRAINING EVALUATION

Fewer major developments took place in the areas of Credentials and Training during the seventies and eighties. However, an in-training evaluation form on each resident was developed, which was to be sent

1978 Long range planning committee is established. Recertification criteria are implemented. Vascular surgery discussions grind to a halt.

1979 Recertification examination committee is established. Vascular surgery discussions with ABS and vascular societies continue.

to the Board office every six months. This, too, was ineffective because the program directors could not be induced to send in the reports. Finally, the program directors were instructed to keep the forms and to submit them with the resident's application for examination.

Not much more progress was made in this area until 1996, when Dr. James Cox, Chairman of the Residency Review Committee, developed a computer program in conjunction with the ACGME, which would allow residents to log in their procedures as they performed them. At any point in training and at termination, the Board would have full and accurate access to the procedural history of the trainee. As of this writing, the program is still under refinement and has not been implemented nationally.

The 30th Percentile

One of the more successful efforts was the 30th percentile figure established as the baseline for operative experience of all candidates. Candidates had to have an operative case load that reached at least the 30th percentile marker of the experience of all candidates applying for examination, or they were not eligible to sit for the certification examination. In part because program directors became conscious of this figure, their residents' operative experience increased steadily. Some of the increase may have been due to increasing numbers of coronary bypass operations and to the ability of the resident to include vascular surgical experience. Still, it was felt that the requirement had a significant impact. The 30th percentile figure finally

DURING THIS PERIOD OF CHANGE AND REDIRECTION, THE BOARD CONTINUED TO CARRY OUT ITS PRIMARY FUNCTION, THAT OF CERTIFYING RESIDENTS WHO HAD COMPLETED SATISFACTORY TRAINING IN THORACIC SURGERY.

reached a point where it was no longer important. Rather, operative experience was to be two to three major cases a week or 125 cases overall, with no fewer than 100 cases in any given year.

From 1983 to 1986, the Board held discussions of developing computer support capabilities. The first system was purchased for the Board office in mid 1980s, and this made it possible to analyze the individual experience of residents in the several areas of thoracic surgery. Areas of concern to the Board were (and still are) congenital heart disease and esophageal disease. On repeated occasions, the Board emphasized that acceptable thoracic training included two full years of training, the last year being at the senior level of responsibility.

THE EXAMINATION EVOLVES

During this period of change and redirection, the Board continued to carry out its primary function, that of certifying residents who had completed satisfactory training in thoracic surgery in an approved program, who were recommended by their program directors, and who met the other criteria for acceptance. The examination was in two parts, a written examination occupying one day followed at a later date by an oral examination. The written examination was first developed with the help of the National Board of Medical Examiners. This was essentially a multiple choice examination that included illustrative material. Because cost was so important, the development of the written examination was placed in the hands of the American

1980 Written and oral examinations are administered separately. Candidate must pass both examinations. A video for the oral examination is produced.

1981 The manual for oral examiners is updated.

Board of Surgery. It was necessary to pass this written examination before taking the oral examination.

A great deal of time and energy was put into the development of a satisfactory oral examination. The manual for oral examiners was updated in 1981. The Board believed that the oral examination measured something different from the essentially cognitive written examination. The goals of the oral examination were:

1. To emphasize problem-solving and not cognitive skills.
2. To allow flexibility for the examiner, that is, examiners were not held to a rigid format, but could expand discussions with candidates.
3. To provide data to allow interpretation of the examination's success in evaluating skills other than cognitive.

Guest examiners were to come from the ranks of program directors and a limited number of two new examiners were selected each year. Great emphasis was placed on training examiners, and video films were developed by John Kirklin and Benson Roe, which proved to be extremely valuable. The Board was acutely aware of the variability in the performance of examiners, and they made strenuous efforts to minimize this by standardized protocols. In 1982, Benson Roe noted widespread support for the use of a mini-conference after every four candidates were examined. A pass or fail decision was made at this conference rather than waiting until the end of the day when fatigue and other elements might make judgment more difficult and inexact.

1982 Certificate of Special Qualifications in General Vascular Surgery is approved by ABMS.

1983 First In-Training Examination is given. Successor to Secretary is chosen.

Frederick Kittle made important contributions to this ongoing effort, and the mini-conference was subsequently implemented.

Some 93% of all candidates who applied for the examination eventually passed and were certified. However, only 79% of residents completing thoracic training were finally certified, primarily because they could not achieve certification by the American Board of Surgery, a prerequisite for the thoracic examination. It is also important to recognize that appropriate appeal mechanisms were included in the examination process under an amendment of the Board's bylaws. These allowed candidates to be immediately reexamined at the same sitting. The appeals applied to the oral examination, but were seldom used. In most instances, reexamination resulted in essentially the same scores that the applicant achieved in his or her original examination.

Much of the apocrypha of the Board's history emanates from the examination process. Denton Cooley came out of an oral examination saying that he had asked the candidate what Alfred Blalock's major contribution had been. The answer was: "He trained you, sir." Of course, Denton passed the candidate.

Physical problems also intruded. One candidate who developed an acute back problem during the examination had to be hospitalized.

A very memorable episode involved a candidate who was pregnant. At the beginning of the written examination, which was being given in Dallas, she announced that she felt she was going into labor. She was

1984 Administrative offices move to Evanston, Illinois. Examinations remain with ABS in Philadelphia.

1985 ABS requests that representative be made full Director of ABTS.

allowed to take the examination in her hotel room. Things went along quietly until the latter part of the morning when she told us that her labor was progressing. Harold Urschel arranged for her to be admitted to the Baylor Hospital. When it came time for her to be taken to the hospital by cab, everyone seemed to have disappeared except the Board Secretary, who had not been directly involved in obstetrics for more than a generation. Nonetheless, off went the patient and the Secretary to Baylor in a taxi. There was not a policeman to be seen on the highway to provide escort, and the trip seemed to take forever. Fortunately, delivery did not take place until she was admitted to the hospital. The sequel is that she delivered a fine boy, and a few days later she completed the written examination. One year later the Board office received a photograph of her son. She later completed the certifying process, and the Secretary received a commendation from the American Board of Obstetrics and Gynecology.

Perhaps the most interesting aspect of the oral examination history was the "missing candidate." During the 1972 examination in Los Angeles, Candidate Number 35 could not be found the day of his examination despite considerable effort. A telephone call from him later revealed that the candidate was in Havana, Cuba, having been aboard a plane which had been hijacked. He finally made his way back to the United States but had to wait another year to take the examination.

Once the examiners were almost lost. The oral examination was to be given at the Chicago State Tuberculosis Sanatorium. Under the

THE FIRST GROUP OF DIPLOMATES TO UNDERGO RECERTIFICATION PROVIDED DATA STRONGLY SUGGESTING THAT MANY OF THEM WERE NOT FULLY OCCUPIED IN THE PRACTICE OF THORACIC SURGERY AND THAT MORE THORACIC SURGEONS WERE BEING PRODUCED THAN WERE NECESSARY FOR PATIENT CARE.

leadership of Hans Ehrenhaft, a taxi full of examiners took off for what proved to be the Chicago Municipal Tuberculosis Sanatorium, many miles removed from the examination site. The examiners arrived just in time at the correct location.

MANPOWER STUDIES

The problem of thoracic surgery manpower was investigated on two occasions by the two major thoracic surgical societies. In addition, a study from the School of Public Health at the University of Michigan made projections about the numbers of thoracic surgeons practicing in the United States in 2013 if present rates of certification were maintained. The conclusions of these investigations suggested that, if 135 thoracic surgeons were certified each year, they would be able to provide approximately the intensity of care provided at the present time. This estimate did not take into account the possibility that rates at which operations, such as coronary bypass, are performed might change.

As part of the recertification process, diplomates were requested to provide information about their operative load. The first group of diplomates to undergo recertification provided data strongly suggesting that many of them were not fully occupied in the practice of thoracic surgery and that more thoracic surgeons were being produced than were necessary for patient care.

> AT THE TIME OF THE GMENAC REPORT, THERE WERE SOME 98 APPROVED PROGRAMS PROVIDING 276 POSITIONS, OF WHICH 133 WERE FIRST YEAR POSITIONS. EMPHASIS CONTINUED TO BE PLACED ON THE QUALITY OF APPROVED PROGRAMS.

On April 20, 1976, the Secretary of Health, Education, and Welfare established The Graduate Medical Education National Advisory Committee (GMENAC) (**Appendix B**). The GMNEAC's Final Report which appeared in April 1981 recommended a 10% decrease in the number of thoracic surgeons trained. The report was immediately criticized for faulty methodology. Although the Board was concerned about manpower, most other studies did not show that we were certifying too many thoracic surgeons. Thus, the Board took no direct action to limit the number of certified surgeons.

The RRC Reexamines Its Role Vis-a-Vis Manpower

The Residency Review Committee for Thoracic Surgery, which had been given a mandate in 1967 to evaluate the training programs in which trainees received their thoracic surgical training, was approached with the idea of managing manpower. At the time of the GMENAC report, there were some 98 approved programs providing 276 positions, of which 133 were first year positions. Emphasis continued to be placed on the quality of approved programs.

The RRC declined to participate in the ongoing discussion of medical manpower in the 1980s by insisting that their purpose was to assure the quality of training programs. They did not believe they should control thoracic surgical manpower by controlling the number of programs or the number of positions in any single program. This was in decided contrast to some other Residency Review Committees from other specialties.

THE RRC DECLINED TO PARTICIPATE IN THE ONGOING DISCUSSION OF MEDICAL MANPOWER IN THE 1980S BY INSISTING THAT THEIR PURPOSE WAS TO ASSURE THE QUALITY OF TRAINING PROGRAMS.

The Residency Review Committee did alter the distribution of training programs so that most of them were associated with teaching institutions. However, the number of available residencies did not decrease at that time.

LONG-RANGE PLANNING AND RELOCATION

A long-range planning committee comprised of Donald Mulder, Hassan Najafi, Herbert Sloan, and Richard Cleveland was appointed to recommend the Board's relocation after Louise Sper's retirement. In addition, this committee addressed the question of the future of thoracic surgery. Questions arose about Board size, adding a member of the public, more orderly rotation of members, representation from regional thoracic societies, and the expanded use of computers in the Board office.

The Committee really concentrated, however, on seeking a new location for the Board. A number of alternatives were investigated, and ultimately it seemed that the Board would require a location with a larger organization which could provide more support. This support was to be administrative but would also involve preparation, scoring, and analysis of examinations. The two possibilities were the American Board of Surgery, located in Philadelphia, and the American Board of Medical Specialties, located near Chicago. With the help of William Maloney and Walter Purcell, these possibilities were evaluated. In 1983, site visits to the Chicago area and Philadelphia were carried out.

THOROUGH CONSIDERATION LED THEM TO RECOMMEND EVANSTON, ILLINOIS, NEAR CHICAGO, AS THE NEW BOARD LOCATION, IN ASSOCIATION WITH THE ABMS.

During these deliberations some of the earlier concerns of the American Board of Thoracic Surgery about domination by the American Board of Surgery arose once more, and old wounds were reopened. After the site visit to Philadelphia, the committee members rehashed all those problems while waiting for their planes in the Philadelphia Airport. Thorough consideration led them to recommend Evanston, Illinois, near Chicago, as the new Board location, in association with the ABMS. However, the Board examination preparation was to remain in Philadelphia because the committee believed that better support for the examination process could be obtained there.

Even as the Board continued to make important decisions about their finances and future, humor would creep into the meetings. To one meeting, Spencer Payne brought a motto for the Board's consideration. In Latin it certainly did not originate in ancient Rome but probably came from the more modern judiciary. The motto was: *Senectus per fidiaque inventutem et artem semper vincere possunt.* (Old age and treachery will always overcome youth and skill.)

The motto was adopted unanimously with enthusiasm. A little later the Secretary was able to provide each Board member with a t-shirt which had the motto emblazoned on it.

In 1986, James Maloney was appointed Secretary Designate, and his tenure overlapped with mine for one year, during which the transfer to Evanston took place.

A 36th Anniversary Album

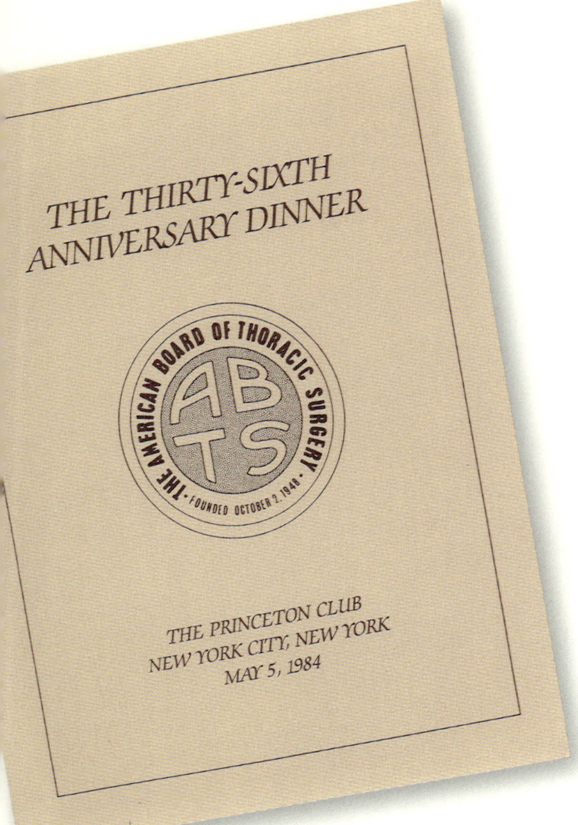

Cover of program from Louise Sper's retirement dinner.

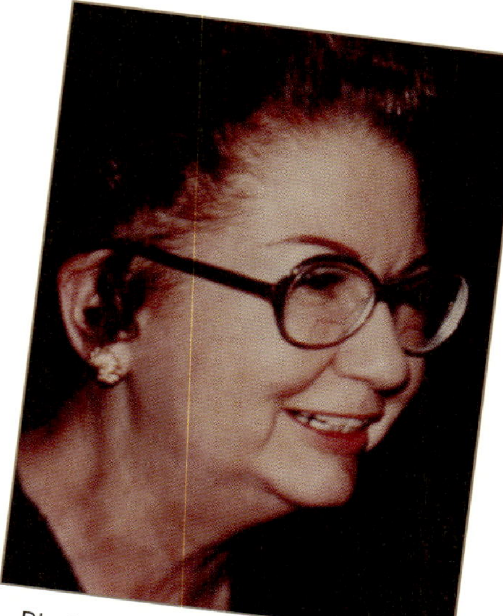

Photograph of Louise Sper as it appeared in her retirement dinner program in 1986.

"The present
joys of life
We doubly taste
By looking back
with pleasure
On the past."

HONORING
LOUISE SPER
Executive Assistant: 1948–1986

As a final gesture, a lovely emeritus and retirement dinner was held in New York City on May 5, 1984, in honor of Louise Sper. Almost all of the living Board members gathered to relive the warm memories each had of his time on the Board and his association with Louise.

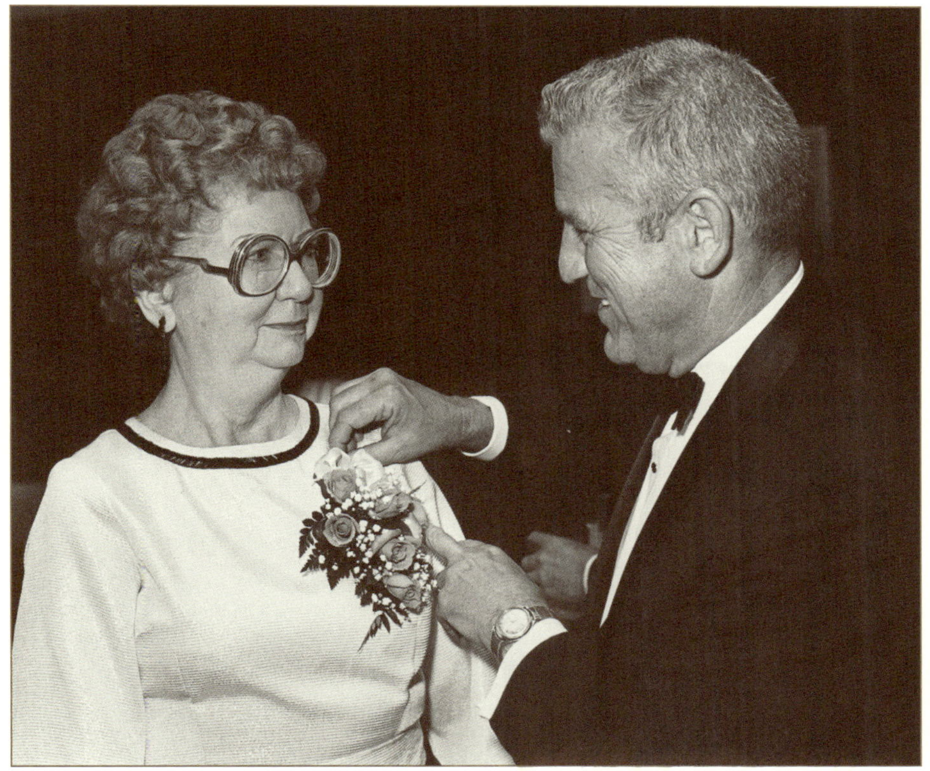

Louise Sper with Dr. Donald Mulder, Board Chairman from 1983–1985.

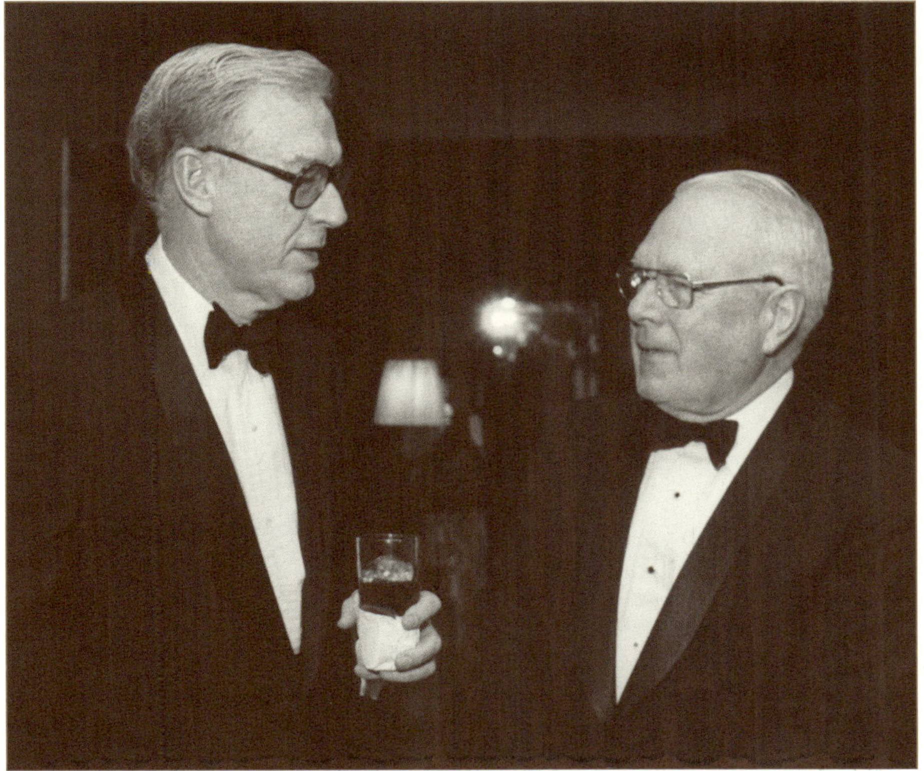

Dr. Tom Ferguson, Board Chairman from 1977–1979, and Dr. Herbert Sloan, Secretary-Treasurer from 1973–1986, chatting at Louise Sper's retirement party.

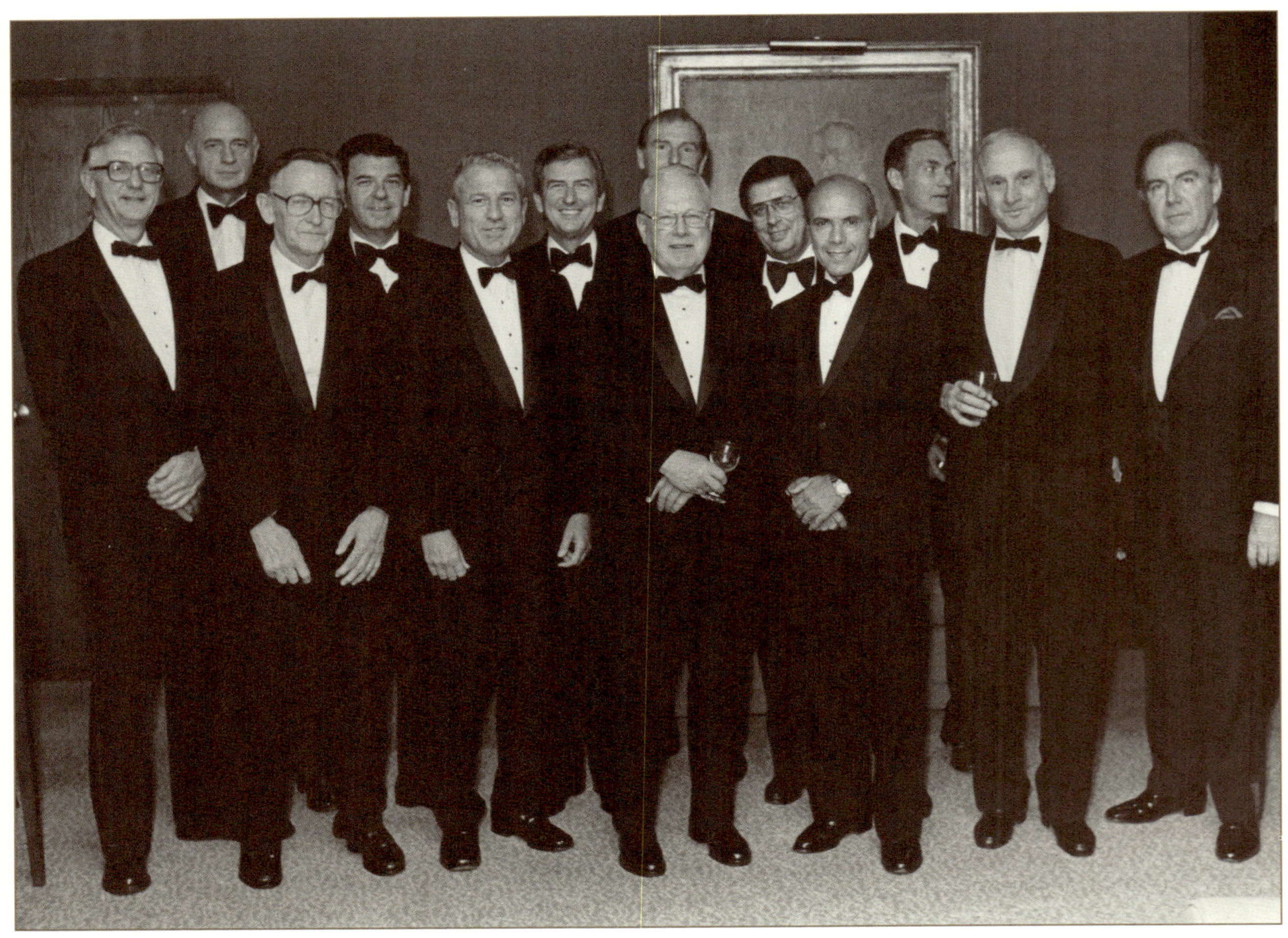

Emeritus members of the Board who attended Louise Sper's retirement party. *From left to right:* Dr. W. Gerald Rainer, Dr. Paul Ebert, Dr. Richard Peters, Dr. John Benfield, Dr. Don Mulder, Dr. Harvey Bender, Dr. Benson Wilcox, Dr. Herbert Sloan, Dr. Richard Cleveland, Dr. Hassan Najafi, Dr. Quentin Stiles, Dr. Hermes Grillo, Dr. Charles Hatcher.

CHAPTER 7

The Maloney Years: 1986–1991

JAMES V. MALONEY, M.D.

1986 Endowment from diplomate solicitation reaches $1,355,736. Endowment fund is segregated and named the American Board of Thoracic Surgery Endowment Fund.

FINANCES, TECHNOLOGY AND PSYCHOMETRICS

Between 1989 and 1991, two forces converged to challenge the Board. The first was a need to justify the reliability of the examination process. It was important to administer examinations that were of equivalent difficulty from one examination to the next.

The second challenge related to the logarithmically accelerating work load of the Board. In previous years, one meeting, or sometimes two, at the time of the annual examination or a society meeting were sufficient. In this era, the Board was responsible for the written examination in Dallas, the oral examination in Chicago, a recertification examination, an in-training examination, and education of Board members in psychometric science. In addition, men who served on the ABTS also participated in the examination process of the American Board of Surgery, the Residency Review Committee for Thoracic Surgery, the Assembly of the American Board of Medical Specialties, and the Council of Board Executives. The ABTS, with only 130 candidates per year paying examination fees, was fiscally ill-equipped to cover related overhead costs compared to other Boards, which examined several hundred candidates each year.

THE AMERICAN ASSOCIATION FOR THORACIC SURGERY AND THE SOCIETY OF THORACIC SURGEONS SAVED THE BOARD FROM INSOLVENCY BY EACH EVENTUALLY DONATING $25,000 DOLLARS ANNUALLY TO SUPPORT THE BOARD'S WORK.

The Endowment Fund

As operating costs rose and as the examination fee could not reasonably be increased further, the anticipated cost of psychometric validation of the written examination and the small likelihood of increasing numbers of candidates to support that work presaged a grim financial future. The American Association for Thoracic Surgery and the Society of Thoracic Surgeons saved the Board from insolvency by each eventually donating $25,000 dollars annually to support the Board's work.

Although it had been with some embarrassment that the Board, under the leadership of Benson Roe, Charles Hatcher, and Harold Urschel, several years earlier had sought the help of thoracic surgery diplomates, they believed embarrassment to be less objectionable than poverty. Thus, the Board sent diplomates a letter suggesting a donation of $300 to establish a capital fund and voluntary *dues* of $50 a year to support operating costs of the examination process. The response could best be described as overwhelming. A large majority contributed and continue to contribute to this day. Most of those not contributing were probably retired or deceased.

As a result of prudent investing and penurious administration, income from the capital fund and from the examination fee have kept the Board in fiscal balance. The Board functions today with the same 2.8 full-time employees in the same square footage as it has for the past 30 years. This was made possible by the generosity of the member cardiothoracic surgeons and by modern technology.

A LARGE DATA BANK OF EXAMINATION QUESTIONS WAS CODIFIED BY SUBJECT MATTER WITH PSYCHOMETRIC PERFORMANCE (PASS RATE, RELIABILITY, AND DISCRIMINATE FUNCTION) FOR EACH TIME THE ITEM WAS USED IN AN EXAMINATION.

Computerization of Board Functions

Glennis Lundberg was appointed as Administrative Director responsible for moving and establishing the new office in Evanston, Illinois, near Chicago. Her technical knowledge together with her master's degree in communications and her personal skills have provided the same kind of admirable service that Louise Sper offered the Board for so many decades.

The computerization of the office begun in Detroit was facilitated by the purchase of a major hardware system financed by the endowment fund. The technical preparation of the certifying examination was brought into the Board office so that the examination could be sent to the printers in camera-ready form. A system for lifetime tracking of thoracic surgeons from the time of application, through examination, certification, and recertification was established. A large data bank of examination questions was codified by subject matter with psychometric performance (pass rate, reliability, and discriminate function) for each time the item was used in an examination. This allowed a complete examination with a predictable statistical reliability with any desired mixture of subject matter to be pulled at will. A separate data bank was generated for formulating the voluntary in-training examination given to residents each year to permit program directors to track the progress of their residents. The experience of every resident in every type of thoracic surgical operation was recorded. This facilitated the work of the Credentials Committee in admitting

1987 Endowment fund finances first major computer system for recording, certification, recertification, retirement, or death of diplomates.

1989 Board decides against accepting candidates outside of programs reviewed and accredited by the Residency Review Committee. Educational Consultant Committee forms to develop new test items.

1991 Position of Examination Chairman is established as permanent member of Executive Committee.

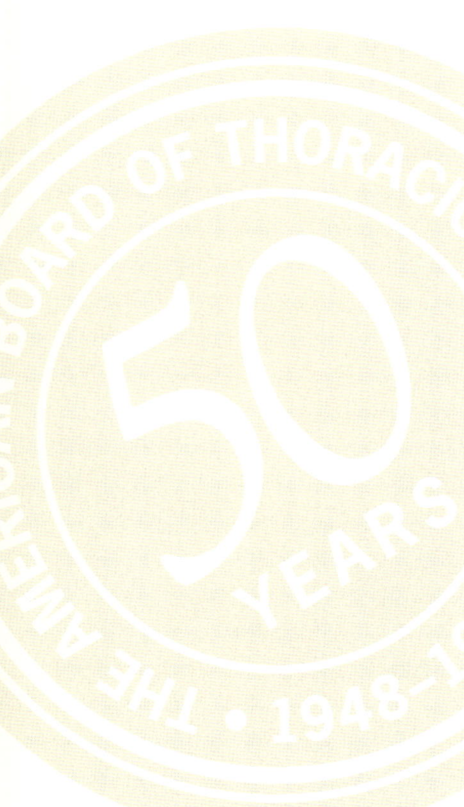

candidates. It further provided valuable insight into the learning opportunity of each residency program.

A Ph.D. mathematician equipped with a laptop computer attended the meetings of both the cardiac and general thoracic examination committees. All corrections and revisions of examination items were completed as discussion was held and subsequently fed directly into the main data bank. This circumvented scores of hours of hand corrections and saved weeks of time for Board members. The computerization of the foregoing administrative functions allowed a several-fold increase in productivity without an increase in personnel. The cost of professional help and computer hardware was made possible by the endowment income so generously provided by the diplomates. Spectacular improvement in the quality of the certifying examination, as measured by the reliability coefficient, resulted. The special contribution of Board members Richard Peters and L. Penfield Faber to this new methodology was substantial. Each consented to serve an extended term on the Board to guide revision of the written examination.

TRAINING ISSUES

Operative Experience

The progression of training concepts from the preceptorial format of the previous era to a true residency program is reflected in the spectacular rise in cases performed personally by residents in the 1980s. The number doubled from a mean of 189 in 1978 to 401 in

IT WAS PARTICULARLY INTERESTING TO NOTE THE PROGRESSIVE RISE IN THE NUMBER OF CARDIAC TRANSPLANTS PERFORMED BY RESIDENTS DURING THIS PERIOD.

1992. Surprisingly, in this era of burgeoning heart surgery, it was the general thoracic cases that showed the greatest increases. Resident experience in other subdivisions of the specialty increased from 20% to 100%.

It was particularly interesting to note the progressive rise in the number of cardiac transplants performed by residents during this period. Although trainees were technically competent, the training programs were challenged to provide in a brief period of time the education in physiology and immunology necessary to practice in this area. Other subspecialty areas share this problem.

The Residency Review Committee has appropriately protected the operative experience of residents by limiting the accredited positions to the number of trainees who can be optimally educated. Post-training fellowships are allowed in those accredited programs only where they enhance the residency rather than compete with opportunities for the resident trainees. Studies have suggested that programs with very large patient loads where the resident is expected to help with the clinical load may offer an inferior education.

Training in Canada

For many years the Board accepted training in Canadian thoracic surgery programs as fulfilling the admission requirements for the certifying examination, provided that the applicant was previously certified by the American Board of Thoracic Surgery. This policy not only

THE UNITED STATES PROFITED SUBSTANTIALLY AS SHOWN BY THE LEADERSHIP ROLE THAT THORACIC SURGEONS TRAINED IN CANADA, BOTH CANADIAN AND AMERICAN, HAVE ASSUMED IN MAJOR UNITED STATES UNIVERSITIES, IN UNITED STATES PROFESSIONAL SOCIETIES, AND IN COMMUNITY PRACTICE.

reflected the warm personal and professional relationships among thoracic surgeons in North America, but made available to Americans some of the finest training opportunities on the continent. The United States profited substantially as shown by the leadership role that thoracic surgeons trained in Canada, both Canadian and American, have assumed in major United States universities, in United States professional societies, and in community practice.

However, a number of asymmetries developed between what was permitted in Canadian programs but was interdicted by policies of the Board and of other organizations involved in graduate medical education in the United States. Thoracic surgeons on both sides of the border were disappointed when the Board ultimately decided to make no exceptions to its long-standing guideline of accepting candidates only from programs reviewed and accredited by the Residency Review Committee for Thoracic Surgery.

The Board and Graduate Medical Education

The unification of the specialty boards and the residency review committees some years ago regularized and separated the process of certifying individuals from that of approving training programs. The American Board of Medical Specialties (ABMS) represented the individual boards and reported to the Accreditation Council for Graduate Medical Education (ACGME). Residency review committees representing each specialty constituency approve training

THE UNIFICATION OF THE SPECIALTY BOARDS AND THE RESIDENCY REVIEW COMMITTEES SOME YEARS AGO REGULARIZED AND SEPARATED THE PROCESS OF CERTIFYING INDIVIDUALS FROM THAT OF APPROVING TRAINING PROGRAMS.

programs and are the essential *raison d'etre* for the ACGME. The ACGME has equal representation of two members from each of five parent organizations, each with veto power: (1) The Association of American Medical Colleges; (2) The American Board of Medical Specialties; (3) The American Hospital Association; (4) The American Medical Association; and (5) The Council of Medical Specialty Societies. Whereas the amalgamation of the constituent organizations under the ACGME is desirable, technical competence in the certification and accreditation process is focused entirely within the ABMS and the residency review committees.

Vascular Surgery

The American College of Surgeons at one time had a cardiovascular committee comprised of cardiac and peripheral vascular surgeons. At that time the College began to recognize that peripheral vascular surgery represented a growing sub-specialty, and they believed they should have their own committee. This done, ACS abolished the cardiovascular committee, and turned over the program responsibility for cardiac surgery to the thoracic leadership, that is, the Board officers and directors. The Regents of the College presented no viewpoint on the cardiac-thoracic dichotomy because it would have been contrary to their view of the way such inter-specialty differences should be dealt with.

In all of the many discussions, both inside and outside the Board, peripheral vascular surgery was considered a part of general surgery.

REVIEW OF THE MINUTES OF THE BOARD'S MEETINGS OVER THE PAST 30 YEARS IDENTIFIES AS THE PRINCIPAL CONCERN THE CONTENT AND DURATION OF RESIDENCY TRAINING PROGRAMS.

This distinction remains to the present time, although that could shift if the conjoint board discussed in **Chapter 6** is approved by the American Board of Medical Specialties.

The American College of Surgeons, for the most part, adopted a "hands-off" stance when it came to different specialties having different points of view. The College's only insistence was that activities such as special experimental programs with three and three residencies be put on jointly by each of the competing specialties. The three and three residencies involved three years of general surgery and taking Part I only of the general surgery boards combined with three years of thoracic surgery.

Training the Thoracic Surgeon

Review of the minutes of the Board's meetings over the past 30 years identifies as the principal concern the content and duration of residency training programs. Repetitive visits to the training issue by the Board usually addressed the following questions:

- Are full training and certification in general surgery a necessary prerequisite?
- Are two years training adequate to encompass the growing subdivisions of thoracic surgery?
- Should basic training in all these special interests be required in all programs, or should specialized training be conducted by a few programs in post-training fellowships?

IN RESPONSE TO THE FEELING OF MANY PROGRAM DIRECTORS THAT RESIDENTS WERE NOT HAVING ADEQUATE TIME AND EXPERIENCE IN SUBSPECIALTY AREAS, THE RRC MADE OPTIONAL THE ADDITION OF A THIRD YEAR TO THE REGULAR TWO YEAR PROGRAM.

- Since practice patterns determined at the time of certification demonstrate that most thoracic surgeons focus their surgical interests sharply, should not training programs reflect this reality?

The possibility of reducing the general surgical prerequisite to three years might well provide basic surgical training for careers devoted exclusively to heart, lungs, and great vessels.

The inclusion of the esophagus in the realm of thoracic surgery makes the consideration more problematic. Certainly a well-trained general surgeon can open and close the chest for access to the esophagus. From half to three-quarters of the first three years of training in general surgery consists of rotations through eight surgical specialties. Does the balance of nine to 18 months on an abdominal general surgical service provide the prospective thoracic surgeon with sufficient experience in an assortment of problems related to esophageal surgery? Does this speak to the Canadian system of separating cardiac and general thoracic surgery training and certification?

In response to the feeling of many program directors that residents were not having adequate time and experience in subspecialty areas, the RRC made optional the addition of a third year to the regular two year program. About a fifth of the training programs extended their training in the face of contrary socioeconomic considerations, as well as the desire of the ACGME to reduce the length of postgraduate training in all specialties. Other programs retained their two year

IN THE PAST 15 YEARS, THERE HAS BEEN A WARM AND CONTINUING COLLEGIAL RELATIONSHIP BETWEEN THE AMERICAN BOARD OF THORACIC SURGERY AND THE AMERICAN BOARD OF SURGERY.

accreditation but continued to send residents overseas or to post-training fellowships in the United States.

The Board made a subsequent survey of resident opinion concerning their reaction to the two types of programs and compared the operative experience of these residents. The subjective response was variable, and no conclusions could be drawn. Surprisingly, there was no difference in the total operative experience of the residents in the two types of programs. The election of the three year program occurred at a time when the Board, with the support of the RRC, was establishing guidelines for evaluating residents' operative experience. Were program directors with marginal case loads extending the training period to achieve case loads that did not threaten the program's accreditation? Or, did the 50% extension in training time provide a better education in the nonoperative aspects of training? These questions are unanswered to the present time.

In the past 15 years, there has been a warm and continuing collegial relationship between the American Board of Thoracic Surgery and the American Board of Surgery in addressing these questions. Creative thinking has been enhanced by having a member of each Board serve on the other. The ABS questioned, as did the ABTS, whether a full five years training in general surgery was necessary for those specialties such as thoracic, pediatric, plastic, and colorectal surgery. Consideration was recently given by the ABS to a four year general surgery program that would provide basic training in general

STATISTICS DEMONSTRATED THAT THERE WERE SO FEW TRAINEES HEADED TO THE SUBSPECIALTIES AND SO MANY TO GENERAL SURGERY THAT THE INDEX CASES AVAILABLE TO THE GENERAL SURGICAL TRAINEES WOULD NOT BE SIGNIFICANTLY ENHANCED.

surgery with, perhaps, some extra time in thoracic surgery. The fifth year would be for those planning on a career in general surgery and would focus on index cases (liver resection, pancreas resection, transplantation, endocrine procedures, for example).

Enthusiasm was tepid on the general surgery side because statistics demonstrated that there were so few trainees headed to the subspecialties and so many to general surgery that the index cases available to the general surgical trainees would not be significantly enhanced. Thoracic trainees were equally cool towards spending their final and best year in general surgical training after the investment of four years in general surgical training already and the desire to be qualified in general vascular surgery.

There is implicit logic in experimenting with changes in curriculum before mandating total revision of the training format. Unfortunately, the experiments thus far in both thoracic and general surgery have not been enlightening. Since the quality of trainees from an institution depends greatly upon its popularity and reputation, the outcome of any experiment is largely determined by the institution chosen for experimental study. Educational psychologists have said for decades that the outcome of education is a function of the quality of student input and that curriculum is of little consequence.

The uncertainty about the training curriculum and the danger of precipitous change based on inadequate data are illustrated by the

A SERVICE CHIEF, RECENTLY TRAINED AT ONE OF THE MIXED PROGRAMS, WROTE, "IT TAKES SEVEN YEARS TO TRAIN THORACIC SURGEONS...IN THE MOST RECENT SEVEN YEAR PERIOD, THE BOARD HAS INSISTED ON THREE DIFFERENT CURRICULA. HOW CAN A SERVICE CHIEF...PLAN IN THE FACE OF SUCH INCONSISTENCY?"

experience of Dr. Tuttle, Secretary of the Board so many years ago. The nature of our specialty changed when cardiac surgery began and chemotherapy decreased tuberculosis case rates by 50% each year. Cardiac surgery centered initially in 13 general surgery programs. The cardiac patients and the tuberculosis patients brought from the sanatoria for operation were on the same general surgical service. The Board recognized the evolution of the specialty and generously accepted trainees from such mixed programs. Soon, however, to regularize education in such non-accredited programs, the Board announced that the 13 mixed programs must establish a separate thoracic service and separate facilities, segregate patients, and have an independent chief of service. The programs complied but some continued to employ six to twelve month thoracic surgical rotations interspersed with the total seven year training program. (This was most often for historical reasons or to permit outside rotations to sanatoria.) Several years later the Board notified these programs that they were disapproved because they did not have the conventional five and two arrangement of general and thoracic training years.

During Dr. Tuttle's era as Board Secretary, a brash young service chief who had recently trained at one of the *mixed* programs wrote to him stating that, "It takes seven years to train thoracic surgeons and in the most recent seven year period, the Board has insisted on three different curricula. How can a service chief rationally plan in the face of such inconsistency?"

THIS WRITER HAS OBSERVED THE BOARD STRUGGLE WITH THE PROBLEM OF THE TRAINING FORMAT FOR 30 YEARS. THE QUESTIONS HAVE ALWAYS BEEN THE SAME, AND THE ANSWERS ALWAYS ELUSIVE.

"Moreover," he complained, "What is the evidence that 'straight' programs are so superior to 'mixed' programs, when the two most recent editions of *The Journal of Thoracic Surgery* show that mixed programs constituting only 15% of the total are responsible for 80% of the advances being reported in our specialty?"

His disapproval was subsequently reversed. Using an age-old administrative gambit, the complainant was silenced by being appointed to the Board where he could, under close supervision, undergo a six year period of reeducation.

Suffice it to say there were no partisan advocacy groups within general or thoracic surgery for any particular change in the current programs. Rather, there was a thoughtful, analytic consideration of the possible public benefit of various options in light of current circumstances. Since the current circumstances, both medical and socioeconomic, are continuously changing, one can be certain that the current format of training in thoracic surgery will evolve over time.

This writer has observed the Board struggle with the problem of the training format for 30 years. The questions have always been the same, and the answers always elusive.

CHAPTER 8

The Fifth Decade

RICHARD J. CLEVELAND, M.D.

1989 A new Educational Consultant Committee is formed.

1992 Board restructures. Thoracic residents matching plan is implemented.

A NEW ERA BEGINS

When I took over the role of Secretary/Treasurer following James Maloney in 1991, Benson Wilcox had just assumed the Chairmanship and John Ochsner was Vice-Chairman. The administrative offices of the Board had been successfully transferred from Detroit to Evanston. Glennis Lundberg had been recruited as the Administrative Director of the Board by Drs. Najafi and Maloney. The addition of Gloria Nance and Jill Grayson completed the office staffing. This new facility and personnel began to provide excellent administrative support for the Board's activities.

In addition, the Board was financially secure due to the fund-raising initiative of Drs. Hatcher, Urschel, Roe and the generosity of the diplomates. Under the direction of Dr. Maloney these moneys were segregated into a separate fund and named the American Board of Thoracic Surgery Endowment Fund. This fund was professionally managed using guidelines developed by Dr. Maloney and approved by the Board. Over the past several years, the Endowment Fund has grown in a conservative and wise manner. The continued generosity

THE GOAL IN ESTABLISHING THE EDUCATIONAL CONSULTANT COMMITTEE WAS IMPROVEMENT OF THE WRITTEN EXAMINATION BY INCLUDING ENHANCED COVERAGE OF RECENT ADVANCES IN THORACIC SURGERY.

of the diplomates of the Board through annual contributions added to the financial stability of the Board.

In 1989, when Harvey Bender was Chairman, a new Educational Consultant Committee was formed. The Board decided that the membership on this committee would be made up of young thoracic surgeons who were making significant contributions to the specialty. The goal in establishing this committee was improvement of the written examination by including enhanced coverage of recent advances in thoracic surgery. The Educational Consultant Committee has matured nicely, and the members of it have contributed significantly to the development of a pool of excellent test items. The Educational Consultant Program continues essentially unmodified to the present time. Several of those who have served as consultants have subsequently been elected to the Board.

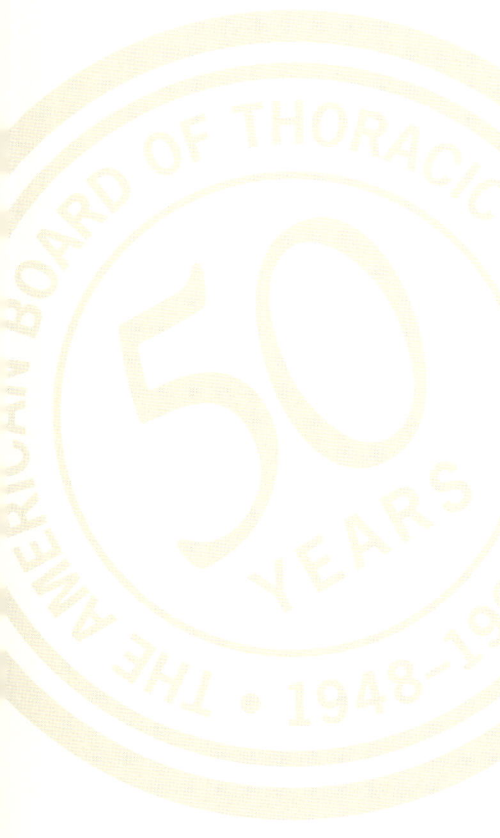

Finally, the Board established a position among the Officers for the Chairman of the Examination Committee. This action reflected the Board's recognition of the importance of the role of the Examination Committee Chairman in accomplishing the Board's mission. That mission continues to be assurance that certification by the American Board of Thoracic Surgery provides evidence that its Diplomates are capable of providing the highest quality of care for those afflicted with diseases of the thorax. The Board had requested that L. Penfield Faber, then Chairman of the Examination Committee, continue in that capacity another two years after his regular six year tenure was

1992 Board modifies bylaws, allowing an individual to serve as Examination Chairman for two consecutive three year terms, as long as his or her total tenure on the Board does not exceed ten years.

1993 Decision to administer the first criterion-referenced written examination in February of 1994 is made

completed. Gordon Murray was appointed as Examination Chair in 1994 and continues in that position as of this writing.

Changes in the Examination

Thus, the essential elements were in place and the Board then undertook efforts to improve its test instruments for certification of individuals who had successfully completed ACGME-approved training programs. Although the norm-referenced written examination had served the Board well in the past, it was clear that modern testing methodology dictated a need for change. Accordingly, the Board engaged Mary Lunz, Ph.D., a psychometrician with a major background in medical testing, to assist in developing and evaluating the criterion-referenced examination. This method of examination required that each test item be benchmarked. That is, for each item evaluated, it was predetermined what percentage of qualified candidates had a high probability of answering it correctly. This would insure a reproducible examination with a high level of reliability of test items that could be reused on subsequent examinations for a predetermined period of time.

In the Fall of 1993, it was decided with some trepidation to administer the first criterion-referenced written examination in February of 1994. Much to everybody's relief the examination was highly successful, and the methodology for the written examination remains unchanged to the present time.

1994 Gordon Murray is appointed as Examination Chair.

1995 Efforts to restructure the oral examination to a criterion-referenced format are initiated.

In 1992 the Board had modified its bylaws, allowing an individual to serve as Examination Chairman for a period of three years and then be reelected to that position for an additional three years as long as his or her total tenure on the Board did not exceed ten years. This important action provided continuity in the examination process. Dr. Faber was elected to that position. Also, the Examination Chairman was added as a permanent member to the Executive Committee so that he or she could participate in this important activity of the Board. When Penfield Faber finished his tenure as Examination Chairman, Gordon Murray assumed these duties in 1994. It is fair to say that, without the leadership of Benson Wilcox and John Ochsner, and the untiring efforts of Dr. Faber, the criterion-referenced examination might not have come to fruition as early as it did or indeed might not have come to fruition at all.

Standing on the shoulders of this successful venture, Gordon Murray, in 1995, initiated efforts to restructure the oral examination to a criterion-referenced format. Although the oral examination has always been recognized as being somewhat subjective in nature, the format was treasured by present and past Board members. Accordingly, any proposed changes in this format would be difficult to institute. Change does not come easily or without anxiety. At the time of this writing the first criterion-referenced oral examination has been successfully administered; however, it will require some further fine-tuning before the Board is as comfortable with this format as it is with the written, criterion-referenced examination.

1996 A significant change in the methodology of recertification is implemented.

The Recertification Process

To the thoracic surgeon, the importance of holding a valid certificate from the American Board of Thoracic Surgery has never been more important than it is today. Indeed the thoracic surgeon's livelihood may well depend on it. In the 1970s, as noted previously, the Board decided to issue time-limited certificates, and a three-part process for recertification was established. This included submission of an application with a practice profile, evidence of appropriate continuing medical education credits, and completion of a self-assessment examination. This format continues unchanged to the present time. What has changed is the number of candidates seeking recertification and the method by which the self-assessment portion of the recertification process is administered.

Recertification has been required of diplomates who received their initial certificate from the American Board of Thoracic Surgery since 1975. Therefore, in the mid and late 1980s, recertification was necessary if the surgeon was to have a valid certificate. In the early days of the recertification process, a significant number of diplomates elected not to be recertified. In fact, up to 20% of the diplomates allowed their certificates to become invalid. The Board decided that, even though a diplomate allowed his or her certificate to lapse, if at some time in the future that individual decided to be recertified, he or she would be declared eligible if appropriate documentation was provided. The situation changed, and by 1993 the number of diplomates

BY **1993** THE NUMBER OF DIPLOMATES RECERTIFYING HAD INCREASED DRAMATICALLY. THE REASON FOR THIS INCREASE WAS THE NEED TO ATTEST TO THE PUBLIC, MEDICAL INSTITUTIONS, AND THIRD PARTIES THAT...THE DIPLOMATE HAD REMAINED CURRENT WITHIN THE SPECIALTY OF THORACIC SURGERY.

recertifying had increased dramatically. The reason for this increase was the need to attest to the public, medical institutions, and third parties that, indeed, the diplomate had remained current within the specialty of thoracic surgery.

Beginning in 1995, individuals who had recertified themselves ten years previously were required to recertify themselves a second time if they wished to continue to hold a valid certificate. About 35% of those individuals recertifying in 1995 and 1996 were individuals who were recertifying for the second time.

A significant change in the methodology of recertification was implemented in 1996. SESATS, which is the instrument of self-assessment utilized by the Board, was published in an electronic version in order to facilitate the process of continuing medical education and, parenthetically, recertification. It is anticipated that, as we go forward, the electronic version will totally replace the pencil and paper version of the process of self-assessment. The initial use of the electronic version has gone extremely well. It is probably a harbinger of methods that may be used in the future for the entire certification process. The Board obviously is indebted to CCCETS for its continuing support of the recertification process.

The father of SESATS was Jay Ankeney who envisioned and initiated the development of CCCETS more than a decade and a half ago. It has provided a valuable instrument both for those who wish to stay

1996 An electronic version of the SESATS, the instrument of self-assessment utilized by the Board, is published.

1997 Carolyn Reed is elected as Director of the Board, making her the first woman to hold this post.

current within the field and also for use within the recertification process. The Board, therefore, is indebted to the past and current members of CCCETS for the development of this fine educational instrument. Going forward, at least in the foreseeable future, the process of recertification will remain in place and will be required by the Board. Parenthetically it should be noted that of the 24 boards who make up the American Board of Medical Specialties, including the American Board of Thoracic Surgery, 22 require recertification at the present time and will do so for at least the foreseeable future.

Restructuring of the Board

Recognizing the continuing changes within the specialty of thoracic surgery and the need for appropriate representation on the American Board of Thoracic Surgery, the members of the Board decided in 1992 that it was time to restructure the Board in order to rebalance its representation. The emerging prominence of the Thoracic Surgery Directors Association (TSDA) brought this into focus, since the Board relies on the program director to attest to the qualifications of applicants for entrance into the certification process. Because the Board did not wish to increase significantly the number of directors for a variety of reasons, not the least of which was financial, it looked at the appropriateness of the distribution of membership from the parent organizations of the Board.

Two major steps were taken at that time. First the position of Secretary/Treasurer, that had traditionally come from one of the

MANY WOMEN HAVE SERVED AS EDUCATIONAL CONSULTANTS TO DEVELOP APPROPRIATE TEST ITEMS FOR THE CRITERION-REFERENCED EXAMINATION. IN ADDITION, THEY HAVE SERVED AS GUEST EXAMINERS FOR THE ORAL EXAMINATION.

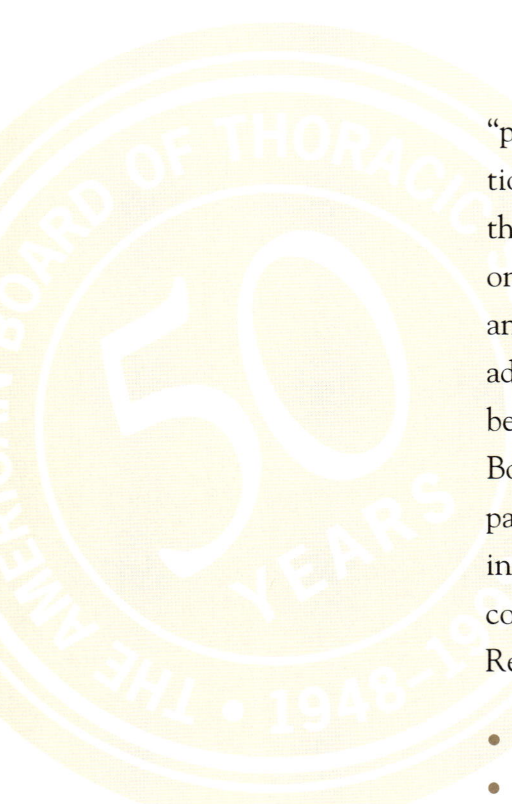

"parents," essentially blocked for a prolonged period of time the election of a younger individual to the Board. Accordingly, it was decided that the Secretary/Treasurer would not come as a representative of one of the parent organizations, but would be elected by the Board for an initial period of five years with the possibility of reelection for an additional five years. This action freed up one position, which could be available for nomination from one of the parents. Secondly, the Board felt the need to have representatives from the TSDA formally participate in the activities of the Board. James Cox was the first individual to be so elected from that organization. With restructuring complete, now in 1997, the Board consists of 17 directors. Representation from the parent organization is currently as follows:

- The American Association for Thoracic Surgery (4)
- The Society of Thoracic Surgeons (4)
- The American Surgical Association (2)
- The American College of Surgeons (2)
- The Thoracic Surgery Directors Association (2)
- The American Medical Association (1)
- The American Board of Surgery (1)
- Secretary/Treasurer-at-large (1)

The Board has also recognized the importance of women within the field of thoracic surgery. Many women have served as educational consultants to develop appropriate test items for the criterion-referenced examination. In addition, they have served as guest examiners

THE MANY ADVANCES MADE BY THE BOARD IN FULFILLING ITS MISSION WERE MADE POSSIBLE BY THE FINANCIAL STABILITY THE ESTABLISHMENT AND GROWTH OF THE ENDOWMENT FUND AFFORDED IT.

for the oral examination. In 1997, Carolyn E. Reed was the first woman elected as a Director of the Board.

As we complete the first 50 years, Marvin Pomerantz has assumed the Chairmanship of the Board. Fred Crawford will serve as Vice-Chairman, and Gordon Murray will continue the duties of Examination Chairman.

Finances

The many advances made by the Board in fulfilling its mission were made possible by the financial stability the establishment and growth of the Endowment Fund afforded it. These funds have been managed conservatively and have grown significantly since its establishment in 1983. Specific amounts have been withdrawn from the Endowment Fund for educational purposes. Some of the activities noted above, such as the consultant program, the development of the criterion-referenced examination (written and oral), and the acquisition of modern computer equipment and software for use in the administrative offices to support the ever-increasing demands are but a few. In addition, the Board has made contributions to several educational programs within the field of thoracic surgery, including the Thoracic Surgery Foundation for Research and Education and the Thoracic Surgery Director's Association for use in curriculum development and an educational conference, for other conferences on curriculum development, and for a research grant to the American Board of Medical Specialties. With the donations to these worthy educational

THE CONTINUED GROWTH OF THE ENDOWMENT FUND ASSURES THE CONTINUATION OF THE BOARD EVEN IN THE FACE OF A SMALL BUT CONTINUING DIMINUTION IN THE NUMBER OF CANDIDATES APPLYING FOR CERTIFICATION.

programs, the Board acknowledges the tremendous support provided by the AATS and STS to the Board during its period of financial travail in the late 1970s. The continued growth of the Endowment Fund assures the continuation of the Board even in the face of a small but continuing diminution in the number of candidates applying for certification. This latter phenomenon is a result of many of the forces acting upon the funding of graduate medical education today that have resulted in a decrease in the number of candidates within programs, as well as the actual number of training programs. Finally, in the discussion of finances it is important to acknowledge the continuing financial support provided by the Diplomates of the Board. Through their voluntary annual contributions, the Board is able to remain operationally and fiscally sound without using any endowment funds for operational purposes. In addition, the Board is cognizant that certification fees are quite high and has adjusted them only by an inflation factor. However, operational costs of the Board exceed this yearly incremental increase.

Acknowledgment

Although the institution of the American Board of Thoracic Surgery has provided the public with assurance of the quality of care provided by those who have been appropriately trained and certified by the Board, I am sure that everyone recognizes that it was not the institution of the Board that has accomplished this, but rather the people who have participated in its activities over the last half century. In the

THE INSTITUTION OF THE AMERICAN BOARD OF THORACIC SURGERY HAS PROVIDED THE PUBLIC WITH ASSURANCE OF THE QUALITY OF CARE PROVIDED BY THOSE WHO HAVE BEEN APPROPRIATELY TRAINED AND CERTIFIED BY THE BOARD.

past 50 years there have been 83 directors of the Board of whom 24 have served as Chairmen. There have been six individuals who have served as Secretary/Treasurer of the Board during that half century. However, there have been just two individuals who have provided the administrative support and guidance so necessary to accomplishing the Board's mission. The late Louise Sper and Glennis Lundberg have served in that role with distinction. Not only past and present members of the Board, but indeed all of the Diplomates have benefited from the dedication and untiring efforts of these two individuals.

CHAPTER 9

Chronology

IMPORTANT EVENTS IN ABTS HISTORY

1925 National Board of Medical Examiners invites AATS to meet in Washington with others to consider establishing a method of certifying individuals in the various specialties of medicine. No action taken by the AATS.

1936 Issue of certification arises again in the AATS. Committee studies the problem of training thoracic surgeons with reference to certification by a national Board. Evarts Graham and John Alexander discuss training of thoracic surgeons. Carl Eggers says special training is necessary but questions if thoracic surgery should be separate specialty.

1937 Committee recommendations presented to AATS and newly formed American Board of Surgery. Decision is made not to establish thoracic certifying board, but to cooperate with ABS in certification.

1940–1945 World War II—Thoracic surgery matures. Surgeons in the field increase pressure to certify thoracic surgeons.

1946 Original certification study committee reappointed after John Alexander encourages Evarts Graham to reconsider a thoracic board. Committee recommends formation of a Board. Stresses need for cooperation with ABS.

1947 AATS approves establishment of affiliate Board of Thoracic Surgery.

'50s

1948 Organizational meeting held in Detroit on October 2nd. Topics discussed:

1. Requirements for founder members.
2. Examination.
3. Application for candidates approved. Office established at Herman Kiefer Hospital in Detroit. Board borrows $1000 from AATS and repays loan the next year. Examination fee set at $100. Louise Sper hired as secretary. Carl Eggers appointed as Chairman. William Tuttle appointed Secretary-Treasurer.

1949 Training requirements established. Examination to be written, oral, and practical. First written and oral examinations administered, practical exam never administered. Competing 'Board' organized in Chicago. Effort dies aborning.

1950 Corporate charter granted by the State of Michigan.

1951 Founder Member group closes.

1952 Stagger system of rotation of Board members begins. First Chairman Dr. Carl Eggers retires.

1954 First discussion of cardiac surgery as part of thoracic surgery. No credit for preceptor training.

1955 First representative to ABS Examination Committee appointed.

1956 Board reaffirms no special certification in cardiovascular surgery. Examination broadened to include more questions in cardiovascular surgery. Directors of thoracic surgery training programs required to have training in thoracic and cardiovascular surgery and be certified by Board of Thoracic Surgery.

1957 Serious difference arises between ABS and BTS on general surgery training necessary to qualify for BTS certification. BTS discusses withdrawal from ABS.

1958 Recorder first used.

1959 First formal representative appointed to ABS.

1960–1963 Emphasis on cardiovascular surgery grows. Term on Board increases to six years from five.

1961 Examination fee raised to $125.

'60s

1963 Mixed training programs no longer approved. Written statement to Advisory Board of Medical Specialties (later the American Board of Medical Specialties) establishes BTS priority of interest in cardiovascular surgery. Pressure from ABMS for BTS to separate from ABS mounts.

1966 BTS participates in a tripartite Residency Review Committee. BTS agrees to accept two representatives from the STS. One year residencies to be eliminated in 1968. Certification of outstanding cardiovascular surgeons who were program directors is discussed.

1967 Residency Review Committee for Thoracic Surgery is established. Program director to sign application attesting to satisfactory completion of training.

'70s

1968 Endorsement of applicant to be required of program director. Applicant must have senior year of residency. Experimental training programs discussed. Discussion of peripheral vascular surgery as part of general surgery and cardiac surgery as part of thoracic surgery. Exam fee raised to $175.

1969 ABMS recommends that BTS become a primary Board. Regional societies will not have Board representation. Exam fee is raised to $250.

Trial training programs to be established. Two more representatives from STS accepted.

1970 AATS and STS make financial contributions. Oral examination restructured with professional assistance. Name change will include American. Office moves to East Detroit. ABS to send representative to ABTS meetings.

1971 ABMS officially approves ABTS as primary Board. 30th percentile ruling adopted. Plan outlined for structured certifying examination to include MCQ and oral examination. Exam fee escalates to $400.

1972 New examination administered; booklet taken and later returned. Self-assessment exam discussed. In-training exam to be discussed with program directors. Oral examination changed to four separate examiners.

1973 Minimum case guidelines approved, bylaws modified. Failed candidates can have hearing.

1974 Self-assessment examination given. 100 case experience accepted for candidates. Candidates must complete approved program starting in 1976. Certificate to be time limited. Committee to examine recertification appointed. Recertification to be required every ten years; concept survives by one vote.

1975 IRS tax exempt classification changes from 501(c)3 to 501(c)6. D.O.'s accepted for examination if certified by ABS and have two years of training in approved program. President of TSDA will attend Board meetings. Vice president of ABTS to attend TSDA meetings.

1976 Trial training programs (3×3) to be phased out. Contributions from AATS and STS continue: $10,000 per year from each for five years.

1977 First operations manual prepared. Committee established to consider requirements for graduate education in vascular surgery. Board office moves to larger quarters. 30th percentile level for operative experience increases from 73 cases in 1974 to 133 cases in 1977. First recording of resident experience. Exam fee goes up to $600.

1978 Long range planning committee to be established. Recertification criteria established. Vascular surgery discussions grind to a halt.

1979 ABTS recertification proposal accepted by ABMS. Recertification examination committee established. Vascular surgery discussions with ABS and vascular societies begin again.

'80s

1980 Written and oral examinations separate. Candidate must pass both examinations. Video to be produced for oral examiners.

1981 Defined benefit pension plan established for ABTS employees. Board requests society contributions to be $25,000 a year for five years. Examination fee raised to $1,000. Certificates valid for ten years.

'80s

1982 ABTS asks diplomates for a contribution of $300 to be followed by $50 a year. Newsletter accompanies request. Successor to Secretary and office relocation considered. Certificate of Special Qualifications in General Vascular Surgery approved by ABMS.

1983 First In-Training Examination given. Successor to Secretary chosen.

1984 Decision made to move administrative offices to Evanston, Illinois, in 1986 with the ABMS. Examinations to remain with ABS in Philadelphia.

1985 ABS requests that representative be made full Director of ABTS.

1986 ABTS representative to ABS now considered full voting member of ABS. Louise Sper retires. Glennis Lundberg is hired as Administrative Director. Endowment from diplomate solicitation reaches $1,355,736. Endowment fund segregated and named the American Board of Thoracic Surgery Endowment Fund. Quarrels about vascular surgery continue.

1987 First major computer system financed by endowment fund for recording, certification, recertification, retirement, or death of diplomates. Data bank of exam questions established, with separate data bank for voluntary in-training exam.

1989 Board decides against accepting candidates outside of programs reviewed and accredited by the Residency Review Committee. RRC votes addition of optional third year to regular two year programs. Educational Consultant Committee formed to develop new test items.

'90s

1991 Position of Examination Chairman established as permanent member of Executive Committee. Psychometrician hired to assisted in development and evaluation of criterion-referenced examination.

1992 Board restructured. Secretary-Treasurer to be elected for five year period. Representative from TSDA formally participates in activities of the Board. Thoracic residents matching plan implemented.

1995 Oral examination restructured to a criterion-referenced format. Second recertification requirement established. SESATS published in an electronic version.

1997 First woman director elected to Board. American Board of Vascular Surgery is formed. Proposal to become conjoint Board with ABS is advanced.

1998 *The American Board of Thoracic Surgery: A Fifty Year Perspective* is published to commemorate the 50 year anniversary of the organization. Two written exams administered, one in February and one in November.

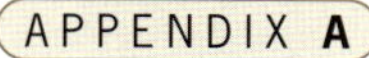
APPENDIX A

Key Points of the Millis Report

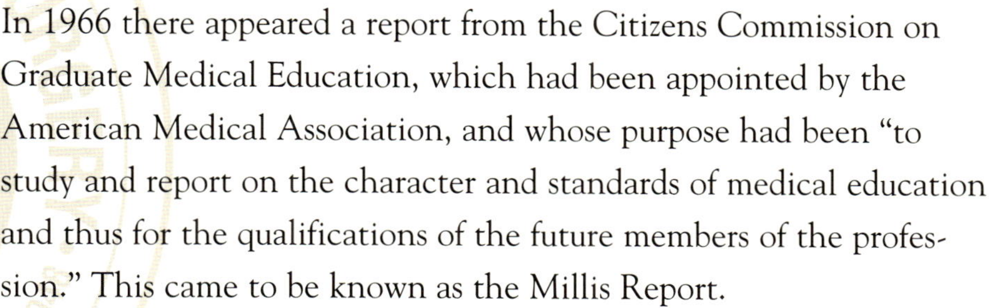

In 1966 there appeared a report from the Citizens Commission on Graduate Medical Education, which had been appointed by the American Medical Association, and whose purpose had been "to study and report on the character and standards of medical education and thus for the qualifications of the future members of the profession." This came to be known as the Millis Report.

In the first decade of the 20th century, a report known as the Flexner Report had resulted in profound changes in medical schools. The Millis Report had a similar effect on graduate medical education.

The Commission looked at graduate medical education carefully and in depth, pointing out both its strengths and weaknesses:

1. Five recommendations related to graduate programs for primary care physicians; all of these aimed to strengthen training for this group.
2. Teaching hospitals should organize their staffs, through an educational council, a committee on graduate education, or some similar means, so as to make its programs of graduate medical education a corporate responsibility rather than the individual responsibilities of particular medical or surgical services or heads of services.

3. The internship, as a separate and distinct portion of medical education, should be abandoned, and the internship and residency years be combined into a single period of graduate medical education called a residency and planned as a unified whole. State licensure acts and certification requirements should be amended to eliminate the requirement of a separate internship.
4. Graduation from medical school should be recognized as the end of general medical education and specialized training as the start of graduate medical education.
5. Hospitals should experiment with several forms of basic residency training, and specialty boards and residency review committees should encourage experimentation.
6. The specialty boards should not increase the required length of residency training to compensate for dropping the requirement of a separate internship.
7. Programs of graduate medical education should be approved by the residency review committees only if they cover the entire span from the first year of graduate medical education through completion of the residency. Programs of graduate medical education should not be approved unless the teaching staff, the related services, and the other facilities are judged adequate in size and quality. Approval should be formally given to the institution rather than to the medical or surgical service most directly involved.

8. Staff members of university medical centers and other teaching hospitals should explore the possibility of organizing an intensive effort to study the problems of graduate medical education and, where feasible, seek to arrange for the development of improved materials and techniques that can be widely used in graduate medical education.
9. A newly created Commission on Graduate Medical Education should be established for the purpose of planning, coordinating, and periodically reviewing standards for graduate medical education and procedures for reviewing and approving the institutions in which that education is offered. There were suggestions about the makeup of this Commission.

Some of these recommendations were adopted in whole, others in part by the various medical specialties. The American Board of Thoracic Surgery approved the elimination of the internship, although this affected the American Board of Surgery more than the ABTS. The creation of the American Board of Medical Specialties stimulated the change to a primary board. Perhaps the major impact of the report on the ABTS was the creation of trial training programs, despite the fact that they were later abandoned.

APPENDIX **B**

Thoracic Surgery Manpower

In 1986 there were approximately 95 approved training programs in thoracic surgery with some 275 positions in the two years of training. On average, 135 thoracic surgeons were certified each year.

The problem of thoracic surgery manpower was investigated on two occasions by the two major thoracic surgical societies.[1,2,3,4,5] In addition, a study from the School of Public of Health at the University of Michigan made projections about the numbers of thoracic surgeons practicing in the United States in 2013 if present rates of certification were maintained. The conclusions of these investigations suggested that if 135 thoracic surgeons were certified each year, they would be able to provide approximately the intensity of care provided at the present time. This estimate did not take into account the possibility that rates at which operations, such as coronary bypass, are performed might change.

1 Brewer, L.A., III, Ferguson, T.B., Langston, H., Wiener, J.M. *National Thoracic Surgery Manpower Study*. Final Report 1974. Los Angeles: Cunningham Press. 1974.

2 Ferguson, T.B. Manpower and services in thoracic surgery. *Ann Thorac Surg*, 1979; 28:4403.

3 Adkins, P.C., Orthner, H.F. The Society of Thoracic Surgeons Manpower Survey for 1976: A summary. *Ann Thorac Surg*, 1979; 28:407.

4 Feldstein, P.D., Viets, H.P. Forecasting health manpower requirements: The case of thoracic surgeons. Ann Thorac Surg, 1979; 28:413,

5 Cleveland, R.D., Orthner, H.E., Bahnson, H.T. et al. Thoracic surgery manpower. *J Thorac Cardiovasc Surg*, 1982; 84:921.

As part of the recertification process, diplomates were requested to provide information about their operative load. The first group of diplomates to undergo recertification provided data that suggested strongly that many of them were not fully occupied in the practice of thoracic surgery and that more thoracic surgeons were being produced than were necessary for patient care.

The Graduate Medical Education National Advisory Committee, established by the Secretary of Health, Education, and Welfare in 1976, advised the Secretary on five national health planning objectives:

1. What number of physicians is required to meet the health care needs of the nation?
2. What is the most appropriate specialty distribution of these physicians?
3. How can a more favorable geographic distribution of physicians be achieved?
4. What are the appropriate ways to finance the graduate medical education of physicians?
5. What strategies can achieve the recommendations formulated by the Committee?

The GMENAC projected a surplus of 75,000 physicians by 1990. By comparison, the Thoracic Surgery Delphi Panel implied that 1,781 thoracic surgeons would be required by 1990. On December 31, 1977, there were 2,165 thoracic surgeons in the United States.

These data raised a hue and cry among thoracic surgeons, particularly among those who had participated in the process. The panelists felt the final number was unrealistic. A number of other *manpower* studies were carried out. By and large they did not support the conclusion that thoracic surgery was overpopulated. At the end of 1994, there were 3,866 actively practicing Board-certified thoracic surgeons in the United States. In 1997, the number rose to 4,117.

Index

A

J

K

L

M

N

O

P

R

S